DR. CHRISTINE OBRIEN

Total Being Reset: A Wellbeing Guide

Cultivating a Heart–Mind–Body Connection for Self–Kindness

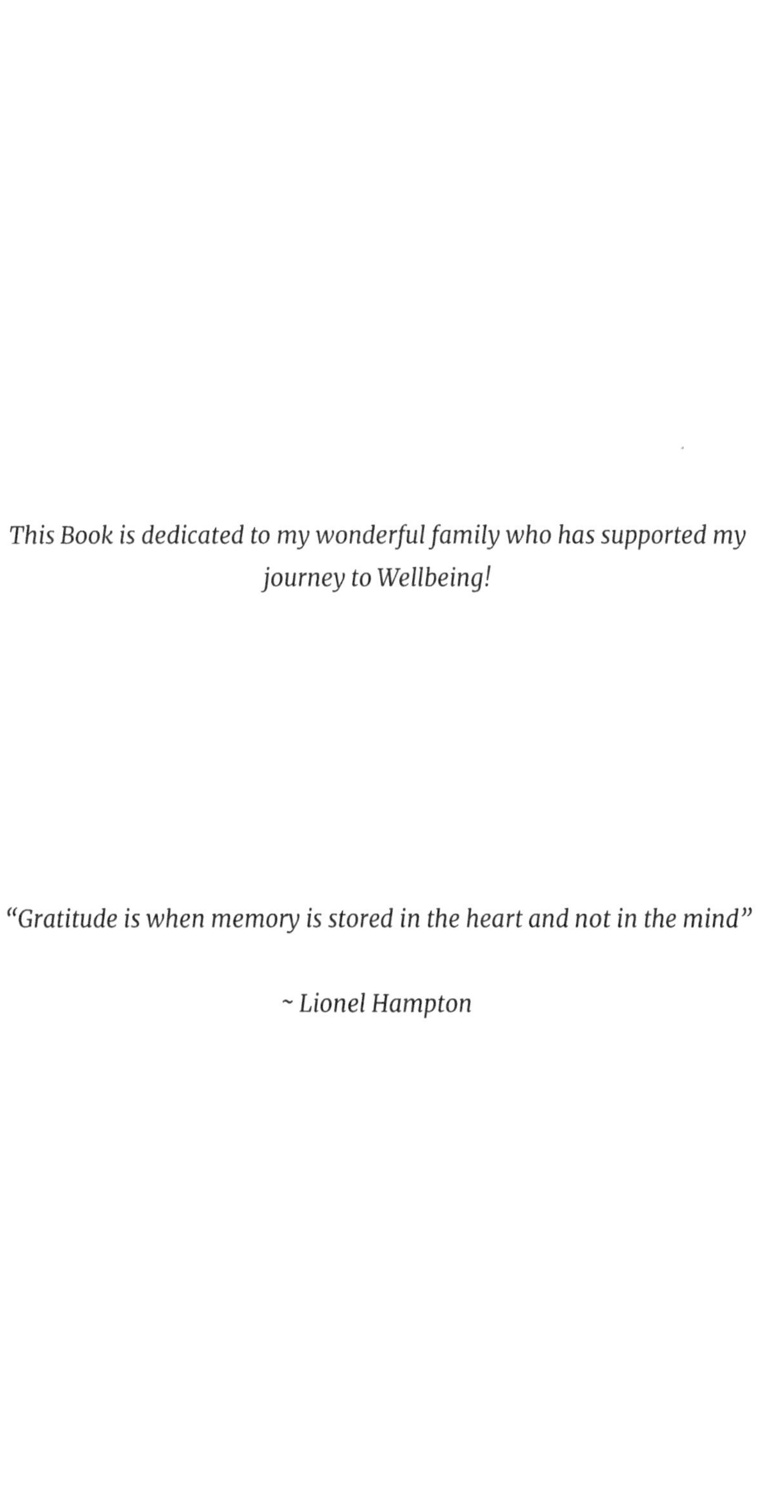

This Book is dedicated to my wonderful family who has supported my journey to Wellbeing!

"Gratitude is when memory is stored in the heart and not in the mind"

~ Lionel Hampton

Contents

Preface   iii

1 Vagus Nerve Activation   1

Conclusion   3

2 Breathwork   5

1. Box Breathing (Square Breathing)   5

2. Alternate Nostril Breathing (Nadi Shodhana)   6

3. Victory Breath (Three-Part Breath or Dirga Pranayama)   7

4. Relax, Release, Reset Breathing   7

5. Heart-Focused Breathing   8

Conclusion   9

3 HeartMath Biofeedback: Enhancing Heart Rate Variability   10

Living the Experience Throughout the Day   11

Benefits of Heart Coherence   12

Conclusion   13

4 Emotional Freedom Technique (EFT)   14

Conclusion   18

5 Yoga Asanas, Tai Chi, and Qigong: Release of
     Fascia and...   19

Release of Fascia: 19

Conclusion   25

6 Sound Healing   26

Conclusion   29

7 Ear Acupressure   30

Conclusion   35

8 Nitric Oxide Dump 36

Conclusion 40

9 Gratitude 41

Conclusion 45

10 Loving Kindness Meditation 47

Conclusion 53

11 Centering Prayer 54

Conclusion 57

12 Ho'oponopono 58

Conclusion 64

13 Awe 65

Definition of Awe 65

Review of Awe 84

Conclusion 84

14 Total Being Reset Conclusion 85

15 Resources 91

About the Author 94

Preface

I have spent my life learning from wise teachers: Thomas Keating, Thich Hnat Hahn, Joh Kabat Zinn, David Steindl-Riest, Deepak Chopra, Andrew Taylor Still, and many more have inspired the layering of principles and practices you will explore in this book.

At the WellBeing Center for Mind Body Health, which I started at a branch of a rural hospital in Western Pennsylvania in the early 1990's, I taught Tai Chi, meditation, nutrition, and center prayer to patients with cancer and other chronic diseases. Now as a trauma sensitive yoga instructor, acupuncturist, HeartMath biofeedback training, Mindfulness Based Stress Management teacher, it is clear that integration and layering of practice was essential to change the lives of veterans with traumatic brain injury, PTSD, moral injury and physical limitations. Patients with cancer, psychosocial issues and autoimmune processes notice the transformative benefits of these practices. Fellow spiritual seekers love learning the epigenetic and generational impact of rewiring mind, body and spirit. After fifteen years working for the VA, I retired from Director of Whole Health at the Cheyenne VA. Total Being Reset LLC is my offering to spark change in individuals, families, communities and the world. Learning from these connections and understanding throughout the years drives my passion to write this wellbeing guide.

1

Vagus Nerve Activation

Activating the vagus nerve can help bring about physical and emotional calm. The vagus nerve is a critical part of the parasympathetic nervous system, often referred to as the "rest and digest" system. Per the Polyvagal theory, activation of the ventral vagus nerve leads to present moment awareness and social engagement thus addressing the loneliness epidemic. Dorsal vagus activation is apathy and that limits ones ability to motive into self-care.

Ventral Vagus Nerve Activation Techniques:

1. **Deep and Slow Breathing:** Engaging in deep, slow breathing techniques such as diaphragmatic breathing or box breathing can stimulate the vagus nerve.
2. **Cold Exposure:** Splashing cold water on your face or taking a cold shower can activate the vagus nerve and help reduce the fight-or-flight response.
3. **Gargling:** Gargling with water can stimulate the muscles of the throat which are connected to the vagus nerve.
4. **Singing, Humming, and Chanting:** Engaging in vocal activities

such as singing, humming, or chanting can stimulate the vagus nerve through the muscles in the vocal cords. Cultures from around the world have for thousands of years.

5. **Laughter:** Genuine laughter can help stimulate the vagus nerve and promote a state of relaxation. A deep belly laugh is good medicine.

6. **Yoga and Tai Chi:** Both yoga and Tai Chi involve movements and breathing techniques that can activate the vagus nerve and enhance parasympathetic activity.

7. **Meditation:** Practices like mindfulness meditation can help activate the vagus nerve by promoting a state of calm and relaxation.

8. **Massage:** Neck and foot massages can stimulate the vagus nerve endings, promoting relaxation and reducing stress. Tough stimulated the feel good chemical "oxytocin."

9. **Socializing:** Positive social interactions and connecting with others can stimulate the vagus nerve and promote emotional wellbeing.

10. **Probiotics:** Consuming probiotics can have a positive impact on gut health, which is closely linked to the vagus nerve and overall mental health.

11. **Exercise:** Regular moderate-intensity exercise can enhance vagal tone and improve overall heart rate variability. Motion is lotion to the fascia and extracellular matrix.

12. **Acupuncture:** Acupuncture and acupressure, especially around the ears, can stimulate the vagus nerve and release acupuncture meridians and fascial restrictions.

13. **Intermittent Fasting:** Some research suggests that intermittent fasting may improve vagal tone and overall wellbeing.

14. **Omega-3 Fatty Acids:** Consuming omega-3 fatty acids found in fish oil can enhance vagal tone and improve mood.

15. **Positive Thinking and Gratitude:** Fostering a mindset of positivity and gratitude can help stimulate the vagus nerve and improve emotional health.

16. **Visualization Techniques:** Using guided imagery or visualization techniques can help activate the vagus nerve by promoting relaxation and reducing stress.
17. **Chewing Gum:** Chewing gum can stimulate the vagus nerve through the act of chewing and swallowing. This stimulates the pharyngeal branch of the vagus nerve.
18. **Spending Time in Nature:** Being in nature and experiencing natural surroundings can help activate the vagus nerve and promote a sense of calm. Awe is the ultimate system regulator as one focuses on something beyond understanding and greater than oneself.
19. **Mindful Eating:** Paying attention to the act of eating, savoring each bite, and eating slowly can help stimulate the vagus nerve and improve digestion as well as focus.

Conclusion

Consider incorporating these practices into your daily routine to help activate the vagus nerve and promote a state of physical and emotional calm. Living in ventral vagus activation to avoid "going dorsal " and to live a full, connected life.

How The Vagus Nerve Affects Organ Systems

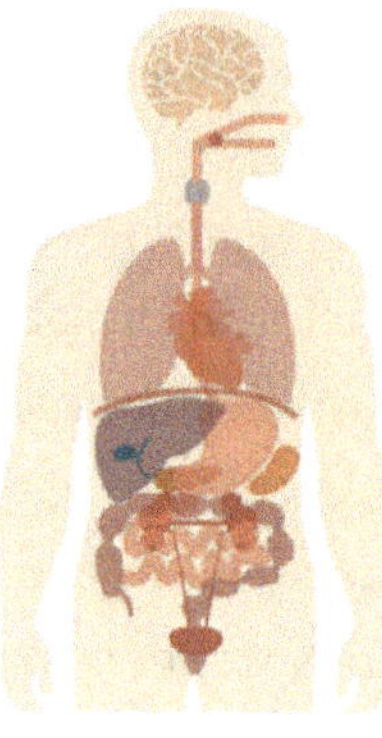

photo source: www.kristenallott.com

2

Breathwork

1. Box Breathing (Square Breathing)

Description: Box breathing is a technique used to calm the mind and body through rhythmic, controlled breathing. It involves equal counts of inhaling, holding the breath, exhaling, and holding the breath again, forming a square or box pattern.

Method:

- Sit or lie down comfortably.
- Inhale deeply through your nose for a count of 4 seconds, feeling your abdomen expand.
- Hold your breath for 4 seconds.
- Exhale slowly and completely through your nose for 4 seconds, allowing your abdomen to deflate.
- Hold your breath again for 4 seconds before starting the next cycle.
- Repeat for several cycles (e.g., 4-5 cycles to start, gradually increasing length of breaths and holds with practice).

Benefits: Box breathing helps regulate the autonomic nervous system, promoting relaxation, reducing stress and anxiety, and improving focus and concentration.

2. Alternate Nostril Breathing (Nadi Shodhana)

Description: Alternate nostril breathing is a yogic technique that balances the flow of energy (prana) in the body, harmonizing the left and right hemispheres of the brain.

Method:

- Sit in a comfortable cross-legged position (or any comfortable seated position).
- Use your right thumb to close your right nostril and inhale deeply through your left nostril for a count of 4 seconds.
- Close your left nostril with your right ring finger, release your thumb from the right nostril, and exhale slowly and completely for 4 seconds through the right nostril.
- Inhale deeply through the right nostril for 4 seconds, then close the right nostril with your thumb, release the left nostril, and exhale through the left nostril for 4 seconds.
- This completes one cycle. Repeat for several cycles, maintaining a steady and relaxed breath.

Benefits: Nadi Shodhana helps calm the mind, reduce stress and anxiety, improve focus and concentration, and balance the flow of energy in the body.

3. Victory Breath (Three-Part Breath or Dirga Pranayama)

Description: Victory breath, also known as three-part breath or dirga pranayama, is a deep breathing technique that helps expand lung capacity and increase oxygen intake. It involves breathing deeply into three parts of the lungs: the lower, middle, and upper.

Method:
Sit or lie down comfortably with your spine straight.

- Place one hand on your abdomen and the other on your chest.
- Inhale deeply through your nose, first filling your lower abdomen (diaphragm) with air, then expanding your rib cage (middle chest), and finally filling your upper chest with air.
- Exhale slowly and completely through your nose or mouth, releasing the air from the upper chest, then the middle chest, and finally the abdomen.
- Repeat this deep, three-part breath for several cycles, focusing on smooth and even inhalations and exhalations.

Benefits: Victory breath helps increase lung capacity, improve respiratory function, promote relaxation, reduce stress, and enhance mindfulness.

4. Relax, Release, Reset Breathing

Description: This breathing technique focuses on relaxing from fight or flight, releasing freeze then resetting into ease.

Method:

- Find a comfortable seated or lying position.
- Take a few natural breaths to settle into the present moment.
- Inhale deeply through your nose and with a slow, long exhale say to yourself: Relax from fight or flight, expelling that tension with your breath.
- Inhale deeply through your nose and with a slow long exhale say to yourself: Release freeze, expelling that tension with your breath.
- Inhale deeply though your nose then with a loud, open mouth sigh say to yourself: Reset into ease.
- Continue this rhythmic breathing, focusing on the body sensations as you continue to relax, release and reset.
- Practice for several minutes, allowing yourself to become more deeply relaxed with each cycle of three breaths.

Benefits: Relax, release, reset breathing promotes physical and mental relaxation, reduces muscle tension, lowers stress levels, and encourages a sense of ease and calmness. It is great to insert between yoga postures, emails, and personal encounters.

5. Heart-Focused Breathing

Description: Heart-focused breathing is a technique that emphasizes breathing with awareness and intention toward the heart center, promoting emotional balance and coherence.

Method:

- Sit quietly in a comfortable position with your eyes closed.
- Place your hands over your heart center, if comfortable.
- Take slow, deep breaths in and out through your heart area.
- As you inhale, imagine your breath flowing into your heart, filling it

with appreciation, compassion, or any positive emotion.

- As you exhale, release any negative emotions, stress, or tension.
- Continue to breathe in this heart-focused manner for several minutes, allowing yourself to feel centered and connected to your heart's energy.

Benefits: Heart-focused breathing helps improve emotional resilience, reduce anxiety and stress, enhance feelings of compassion and connection, and promote overall wellbeing and heart coherence.

Conclusion

These breathing practices can be powerful tools for cultivating mindfulness, reducing stress, and enhancing overall wellbeing when practiced regularly and frequently with intention to rewire the renewing emotions and physical sensations creating an upgrade in whole person integration.

3

HeartMath Biofeedback: Enhancing Heart Rate Variability

Heart Rate Variability (HRV) refers to the variation in the time interval between heartbeats. A healthy heart doesn't beat like a metronome; there are slight variations in the time interval between beats. Higher HRV is associated with better health and fitness, while lower HRV is linked to stress, fatigue, and various health problems.

How HeartMath Biofeedback Works to Enhance HRV:

HeartMath biofeedback is a technique designed to improve HRV by training individuals to shift their physiological and emotional state towards coherence. It involves the following steps:

Heart-Focused Breathing:

- Heart-focused breathing is a technique where you consciously breathe deeply and rhythmically through the heart area. This technique helps synchronize the heart rhythm and activate the parasympathetic nervous system, promoting relaxation and reducing stress.

Feelings of Love, Care, and Appreciation:

- HeartMath emphasizes generating positive emotions such as love, care, and appreciation. When you focus on these feelings towards someone, something, or someplace, it creates a coherent heart rhythm pattern and enhances HRV.

Awe Experience:

- Experiencing awe, such as holding a sleeping child or being in nature, can induce goosebumps and activate a profound, renewing emotional response. This emotional state is associated with heart coherence, where the heart rhythm becomes coherent and harmonious.

Living the Experience Throughout the Day

To integrate the benefits of heart coherence into your daily life, follow these steps:

Morning Practice:

- Start your day with heart-focused breathing and cultivate feelings of love, care, and appreciation during your morning routine. This sets a positive tone for the day and enhances emotional resilience.

Midday Break:

- Take a break to engage in an awe experience, such as spending time in nature or connecting with loved ones. Notice the sensations in your body, including any goosebumps or feelings of warmth and connection.

Evening Reflection:

- Before bed, reflect on moments of heart coherence throughout the day. Recall instances where you felt deeply connected and appreciative. This reflection reinforces positive emotional states and supports relaxation.

Benefits of Heart Coherence

Personal Benefits:

- Enhanced emotional resilience and stress reduction.
- Improved cardiovascular health and regulation of blood pressure.
- Enhanced cognitive function and mental clarity.
- Better sleep quality and overall wellbeing.
- Interpersonal Benefits:
- Improved communication and empathy in relationships.
- Strengthened emotional connections and intimacy.
- Reduced conflict and increased cooperation.

Electromagnetic Field and Connection with Earth's Field:

A person in a coherent state emits a coherent electromagnetic field from the heart, which is measurable several feet away from the body. This electromagnetic field interacts with the Earth's magnetic field, potentially creating a harmonious resonance that promotes overall health and wellbeing.

Conclusion

Incorporating HeartMath biofeedback and practices like heart-focused breathing, feelings of love and appreciation, and awe experiences into your daily routine can significantly enhance heart coherence and improve overall health. By cultivating positive emotions and connecting with the heart's wisdom, you benefit yourself and also contribute to a more harmonious and interconnected world. Embrace these practices with consistency and intention to foster resilience, compassion, and wellbeing in your life and beyond.

4

Emotional Freedom Technique (EFT)

Emotional Freedom Technique (EFT), often referred to as "tapping," is an alternative therapy that combines elements of acupressure and positive affirmation to address both emotional and physical issues.

The Basics of EFT

EFT is based on the premise that negative emotions are linked to disturbances in the body's energy system. By tapping on specific meridian points (similar to acupuncture points) while focusing on a particular issue and using positive affirmations, we aim to restore balance in the energy system, thereby alleviating emotional distress and improving overall wellbeing.

How EFT Works

Identify the Issue: The first step in EFT is to pinpoint the specific issue you want to address. This could be a negative emotion, physical pain, or a limiting belief.

Establish a Setup Statement: Create a setup statement that acknowledges the issue while also affirming self-acceptance. This typically follows the format: "Even though I have [this issue], I deeply and completely accept myself."

Tapping Sequence: Tap on specific meridian points on the body while repeating a reminder phrase related to the issue. The commonly used meridian points include:

- The top of the head
- The beginning of the eyebrow
- The side of the eye
- Under the eye
- Under the nose
- The chin point
- The beginning of the collarbone
- The side of the hand (Karate chop point)
- Under the arm

Tapping Points

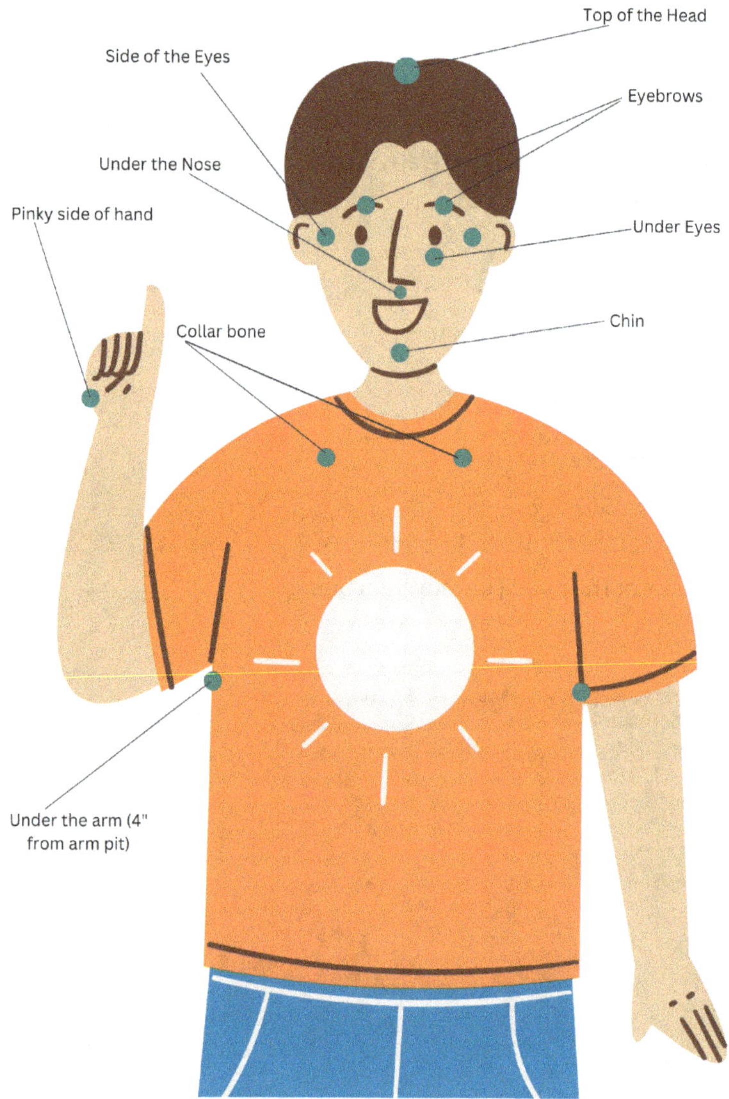

Repeat and Adjust: Perform several rounds of tapping, reassessing the intensity of the issue after each round. Adjust the statements and tapping sequence as necessary to continue addressing the issue.

Combining Acupressure and Positive Affirmation

EFT combines acupressure and positive affirmation to create a synergistic effect:

Acupressure: Tapping on specific meridian points is believed to stimulate the flow of energy (Qi) in the body, similar to the principles of acupuncture and acupressure. This helps to release blockages and restore balance in the energy system.

Positive Affirmation: Using positive affirmations during the tapping process helps to reframe negative thoughts and emotions, fostering a sense of self-acceptance and positive outlook.

Higher Energy Feeling States and Connection

EFT practitioners often emphasize the importance of focusing on higher energy feeling states, such as love, gratitude, and peace. By doing so, individuals may enhance their ability to connect with universal energy or source energy, which is believed to be a limitless and supportive force.

Higher Energy Feeling States: Emotions like love, joy, and gratitude are considered higher vibrational states. Focusing on these emotions can help to raise an individual's overall energy frequency, promoting a sense of wellbeing and connection to something greater than themselves.

Connection with Universal Energy: EFT can facilitate a deeper connection with universal energy or source energy by helping individuals release negative emotions and limiting beliefs. This process is thought to open up pathways for receiving guidance, support, and inspiration from a higher source.

Benefits of EFT

Emotional Healing: EFT is commonly used to address issues such as anxiety, depression, trauma, and phobias by helping individuals process and release negative emotions.

Physical Healing: Many practitioners believe that by resolving emotional issues, EFT can also alleviate physical symptoms and pain that are linked to emotional distress.

Enhanced Wellbeing: Regular practice of EFT can promote overall emotional resilience, a positive mindset, and a sense of calm and balance.

Conclusion

EFT is a versatile and user-friendly technique that can be practiced alone or with the guidance of a trained EFT practitioner. While scientific research on EFT is still evolving, many individuals report significant benefits from incorporating it into their wellness routines.

5

Yoga Asanas, Tai Chi, and Qigong: Release of Fascia and Increased Flow in the Extracellular Matrix

Release of Fascia:

Yoga Asanas: Yoga involves a series of postures (asanas) that stretch and strengthen the muscles, but also apply gentle tension to the fascial tissues. Fascia is a connective tissue that surrounds muscles, bones, and organs, providing structure and support. Through various yoga poses, fascial adhesions can be released, improving flexibility and range of motion.

Tai Chi and QiGong: These Chinese movement practices also emphasize fluid, circular movements that gently stretch and release fascial tissues. By moving the body in a slow and deliberate manner, they help to unwind tension in the fascia, promoting better mobility and circulation.

Enhanced Flow in the Extracellular Matrix

The extracellular matrix (ECM) is a complex network of proteins, glyco-proteins, and other molecules that surround cells and provide structural support. Both yoga and practices like tai chi and qigong stimulate the ECM by promoting movement and fluidity.

Yoga: Asanas create micro-movements and stretches that encourage the flow of interstitial fluid within the ECM. This fluid carries nutrients, hormones, and neurotransmitters to cells and tissues, supporting overall health and function.

Tai Chi and QiGong: These practices promote the circulation of Qi (life energy) through the meridian pathways of the body. The movements help to open energy blockages and stimulate the flow of blood and lymphatic fluid in the ECM, enhancing cellular communication and metabolic processes.

Neurotransmitters, Hormones, Nutrients, and Circulation

Yoga: Asanas can stimulate the endocrine system, which regulates hormone production and secretion. Certain poses, such as inversions, can improve blood circulation to the brain, enhancing neurotransmitter function and cognitive clarity.

Tai Chi and QiGong: These practices are believed to balance the autonomic nervous system, which influences the release of neurotransmitters and hormones. Improved circulation and oxygenation through gentle movement support overall cellular health and function.

Concepts by Andrew Taylor Still and Buckminster Fuller

Andrew Taylor Still: Fascia as the Soul:

Andrew Taylor Still, the founder of osteopathy, proposed that the fascia is central to health and vitality. He believed that disruptions in the fascial network could impair the flow of vital fluids and energy throughout the body, leading to disease.

According to Still, the fascia acts as a conduit for the flow of life force (sometimes referred to as "soul") within the body. Maintaining the health and integrity of the fascia through movement, manual therapy, and fascia release techniques is essential for optimal health and wellbeing.

Buckminster Fuller: Tensegrity as Balance and Support:

Buckminster Fuller, an architect and inventor, introduced the concept of "tensegrity" (tensional integrity) in structures. Tensegrity refers to a structural system where tensional and compressive forces interact to maintain balance and stability.

In the context of the human body, tensegrity suggests that the skeletal system (compression) and the fascial network (tension) work together to provide support and maintain structural integrity. The fascia, with its tensile strength and elasticity, plays a crucial role in distributing forces and maintaining alignment in response to movement and gravity.

Tensegrity principles are reflected in the dynamic balance and flexibility observed in practices like yoga, tai chi, and chi gong. These movements promote optimal alignment, flexibility, and strength by engaging the fascial network and skeletal system in a harmonious relationship.

The principles of tensegrity apply to essentially every detectable size scale of the body from nucleus > cells > tissues> organs > systems > people.

As a tensegrity structure, fascia is in a constant state of dynamic balanced tension as fascia moves as a unit within this tensegrity system down to the microscopic level. Injury to fascia locally at one body region will be carried throughout the whole fascial network.

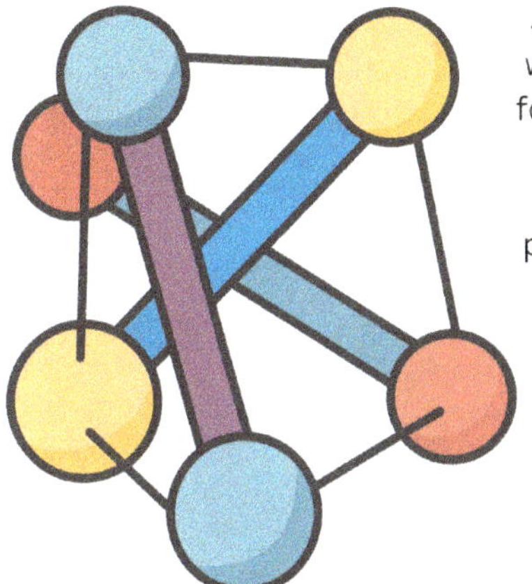

Just like a child's Skwish toy, which bends by distributing a force through the strings, your fascia plays the same role throughout the body, promoting optimal alignment, flexibility, and strength.

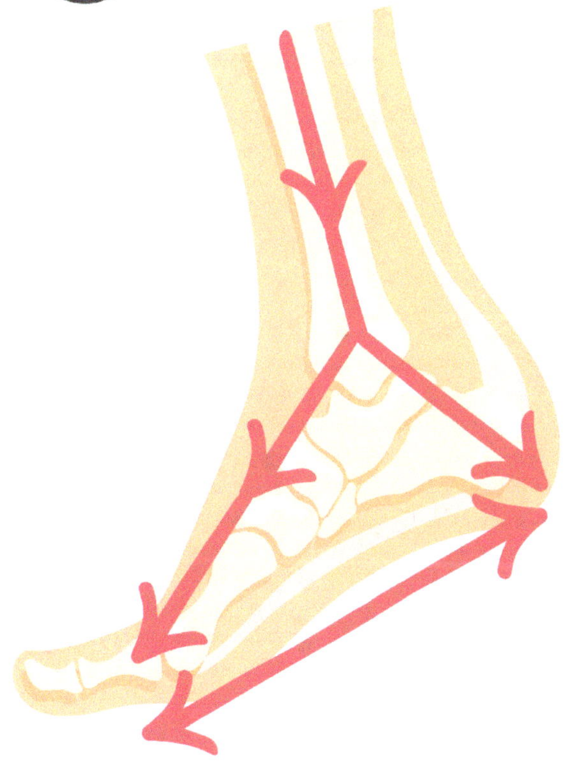

Myofascial lines

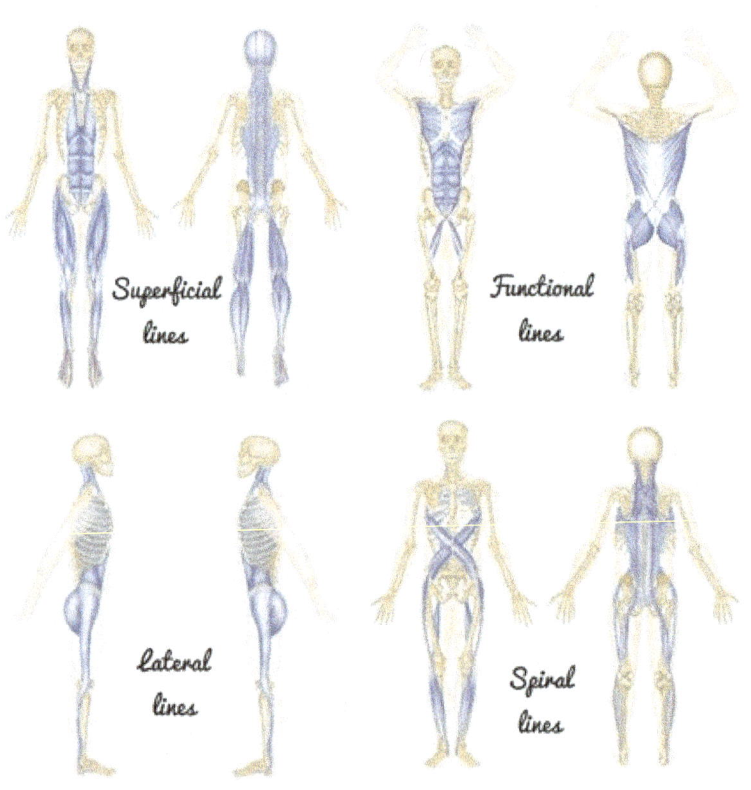

Image from Anatomy Trains by Thomas W Myers 2009.

Conclusion

In summary, yoga asanas, tai chi, and qigong stimulate the release of fascia and enhance flow within the extracellular matrix. These practices promote the circulation of neurotransmitters, hormones, and nutrients, supporting overall health and vitality. Andrew Taylor Still's concept of fascia as the soul emphasizes the integral role of fascia in maintaining vitality, while Buckminster Fuller's concept of tensegrity underscores the importance of structural integrity and balance in the human system. Together, these concepts highlight the interconnectedness of movement, fascial health, and holistic wellbeing in practices that promote physical, mental, and energetic harmony.

6

Sound Healing

Sound Healing using crystal bowls, also known as crystal bowl therapy or sound bath therapy, involves using specific frequencies and vibrations produced by crystal singing bowls to facilitate healing and balance in the body, mind, and spirit. Here's how this practice creates heart coherence, resonance, and attunement with oneself and others:

Mechanism of Crystal Bowl Sound Healing

Resonance with Chakra/Energy Centers:

Crystal bowls are often tuned to specific frequencies that correspond to the energy centers or chakras of the body. Each chakra is associated with particular frequencies and qualities. For example, the heart chakra is often associated with the frequency of 432 Hz.

When a crystal bowl is struck or played, it emits a pure tone that resonates with the corresponding chakra. This resonance is believed to stimulate and balance the energy flow within the chakra, promoting harmony and wellbeing.

Vibration and Energy Flow:

Sound waves produced by crystal bowls travel through the body as vibrations. These vibrations can penetrate deeply into tissues, organs, and energy pathways (meridians), affecting the subtle energy system of the body.

By resonating with the chakras and energy centers, crystal bowl sound vibrations help to clear blockages, release stagnant energy, and restore the natural flow of energy throughout the body.

Heart Coherence and Resonance:

The heart is not only a physical organ but also considered a center of emotional and energetic coherence. Crystal bowl sound healing can entrain the heart to coherent rhythms, promoting emotional balance, and reducing stress and anxiety.

As the vibrations of crystal bowls resonate with the heart chakra, they can induce feelings of peace, love, and compassion. This coherence in the heart's electromagnetic field synchronizes with brain waves, promoting a state of relaxation and harmony.

Attunement with Self and Others:

Sound healing with crystal bowls can facilitate a deep sense of connection and attunement with oneself. As the vibrations penetrate the body and mind, individuals may experience a heightened awareness of their inner state and emotions.

When practiced in groups or with others, crystal bowl sound healing can create a collective resonance. The harmonizing vibrations foster a sense of unity and interconnectedness among participants, promoting empathy, understanding, and mutual support.

This shared experience of resonance and attunement can enhance social coherence and strengthen interpersonal relationships.

Benefits of Crystal Bowl Sound Healing

- **Stress Reduction and Relaxation:** Promotes relaxation and reduces stress by calming the nervous system.
- **Emotional Release and Healing:** Facilitates emotional release and supports emotional healing by clearing energetic blockages.
- **Enhanced Mental Clarity:** Improves focus, concentration, and mental clarity by harmonizing brain waves.
- **Physical Wellbeing:** Supports physical healing processes by enhancing circulation, reducing pain, and improving sleep quality.
- **Spiritual Connection:** Deepens spiritual awareness and connection by facilitating meditation and inner exploration.

Practical Considerations

Sessions: Crystal bowl sound healing sessions can be conducted individually or in group settings. Participants typically lie down or sit comfortably while experiencing the vibrations of the bowls. If sessions are unavailable or inaccessible, you can always find videos on youtube.

Frequency: Regular sessions may be beneficial to maintain energetic balance and support overall wellbeing.

Integration: Crystal bowl sound healing can complement other holistic practices such as meditation, yoga, and energy work.

Conclusion

Crystal bowl sound healing harnesses the power of vibrations and resonance to create heart coherence, emotional balance, and attunement with self and others. By harmonizing with the frequencies of chakras and energy centers, this practice supports the free flow of energy within and around the human system, fostering holistic healing and transformation. Consider listening to a youtube sound healing as you work at your computer or as you sleep.

7

Ear Acupressure

Ear acupressure, also known as auriculotherapy or ear reflexology, is based on the principle that the ear is a microsystem of the entire body. This means that specific points on the ear correspond to different organs, systems, and parts of the body. By stimulating these points through acupressure techniques, it is believed that one can influence and treat various health issues throughout the body.

Microsystem Concept:

The ear contains numerous acupressure points that correspond to specific areas of the body, similar to how reflexology maps the feet or hands. Stimulating these points is believed to promote balance and healing in corresponding organs, systems, and body parts.

Stimulation Techniques:

Acupressure involves applying gentle pressure to specific points on the ear using fingers, thumbs, or specialized tools. Techniques may include massaging, pressing, or rotating the points to stimulate them.

Benefits:

Ear acupressure is used to alleviate pain, reduce stress, improve circu-lation, enhance immune function, and promote overall wellbeing. It is often used as a complementary therapy alongside with body acupuncture and conventional medical treatments.

Ear Acupressure Points and Their Corresponding Areas

Below is a general description of some key ear acupressure points and their locations, along with their corresponding areas of the body:

Ear Lobe:

- The ear lobe is often associated with the head and face region, including the eyes, nose, and mouth as well as the brain.

Center of the Ear (Point Zero):

- Located in the upper center of the ear, Point Zero stimulates the internal organs and the vagus nerve.

Triangular Fossa Notch:

- The triangular fossa is a point that corresponds to the hips and knees. Stimulating this point may help alleviate pain and discomfort in these areas.
- Shen Men is a master point to bring relaxation to the whole body.

Sacral Point:

- This point corresponds to the sacral region of the spine, influencing lower back pain and pelvic issues.

Spine Points:

- The spine point runs along the outer edge of the ear, corresponding to the entire spine from cervical to lumbar regions.

Allergy Point:

- Located on the outer ear near the top, this point is believed to help alleviate allergy symptoms and strengthen the immune system.

Fingers, Hands, Forearm, Elbow, Shoulders:

- Various points on the outer ear correspond to these areas, providing relief for pain, stiffness, and tension.

Pressure Points on the Ear (Diagram)

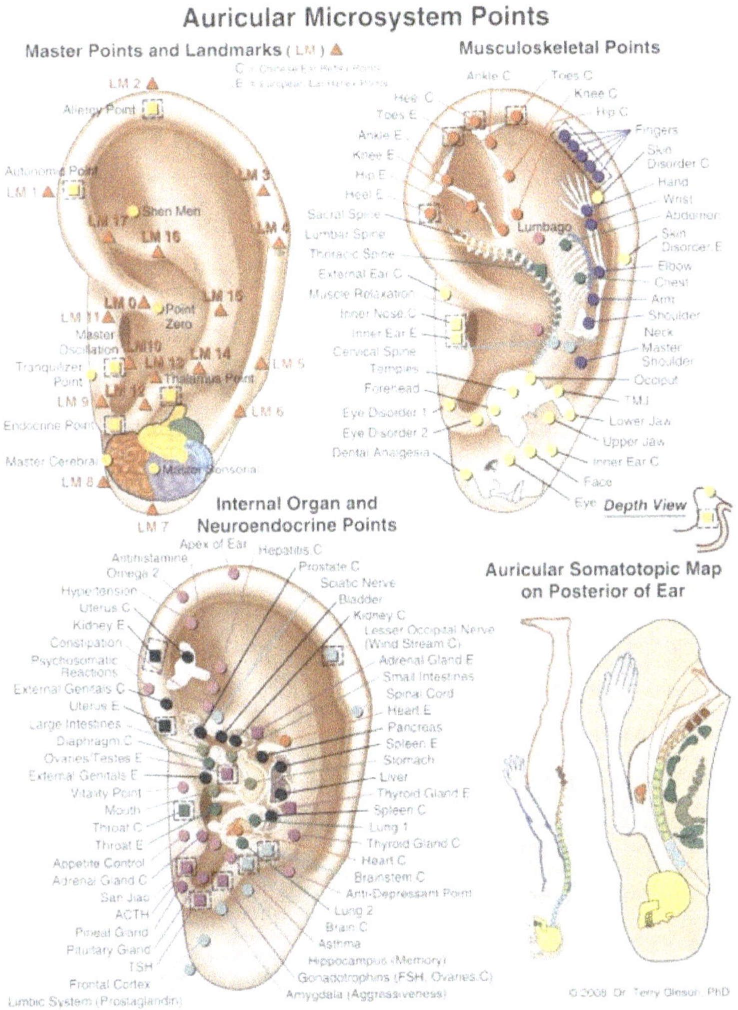

Auricular Microsystem Points

Master Points and Landmarks (LM) ▲

C = Chinese Ear Reflex Points
E = European Ear Reflex Points

LM 2 ▲
Allergy Point
Autonomic Point
LM 1 ▲
LM 17
Shen Men
LM 16
LM 3
LM 4
LM 0 ▲
Point Zero
LM 11 ▲
LM 15
Master Oscillation
LM 10
LM 14
Tranquilizer Point
LM 13
LM 12
Thalamus Point
LM 5
LM 9
Endocrine Point
LM 6
Master Cerebral
Master Sensorial
LM 8 ▲
LM 7

Musculoskeletal Points

Ankle C
Toes C
Heel C
Knee C
Toes E
Hip C
Ankle E
Fingers
Knee E
Skin Disorder C
Hip E
Hand
Heel E
Wrist
Sacral Spine
Abdomen
Lumbar Spine
Lumbago
Skin Disorder E
Thoracic Spine
Elbow
External Ear C
Chest
Muscle Relaxation
Arm
Inner Nose C
Shoulder
Inner Ear E
Neck
Cervical Spine
Master Shoulder
Temples
Occiput
Forehead
TMJ
Eye Disorder 1
Lower Jaw
Eye Disorder 2
Upper Jaw
Dental Analgesia
Inner Ear C
Face
Eye
Depth View

Internal Organ and Neuroendocrine Points

Apex of Ear
Hepatitis C
Antihistamine
Omega 2
Prostate C
Sciatic Nerve
Hypertension
Bladder
Uterus C
Kidney C
Kidney E
Lesser Occipital Nerve
Constipation
(Wind Stream C)
Psychosomatic Reactions
Adrenal Gland E
External Genitals C
Small Intestines
Uterus E
Spinal Cord
Large Intestines
Heart E
Diaphragm C
Pancreas
Ovaries/Testes E
Spleen E
External Genitals E
Stomach
Vitality Point
Liver
Mouth
Thyroid Gland E
Throat C
Spleen C
Throat E
Lung 1
Appetite Control
Thyroid Gland C
Adrenal Gland C
Heart C
San Jiao
Brainstem C
ACTH
Anti-Depressant Point
Pineal Gland
Lung 2
Pituitary Gland
Brain C
TSH
Asthma
Frontal Cortex
Hippocampus (Memory)
Limbic System (Prostaglandin)
Gonadotrophins (FSH, Ovaries C)
Amygdala (Aggressiveness)

Auricular Somatotopic Map on Posterior of Ear

© 2008 Dr. Terry Oleson, PhD

Effectiveness in Treating the Entire System

Holistic Approach: Ear acupressure takes a holistic approach by addressing physical, emotional, and energetic imbalances through targeted stimulation of specific points.

Comprehensive Treatment: By systematically stimulating points from the ear lobe to the top of the ear, one can address a wide range of health issues including pain, inflammation, digestive problems, and emotional stress.

- Start by massaging the ear lobe, move index finger into ear near ear canal massaging the areas above and below point zero to stimulate the internal organs.
- Now, press on Shen Men, hip and knee points.
- Move to the top of the ear massaging the allergy point and migrate with constant connection of the fingers down the outer aspect of the ear massaging the fingers, arms, shoulder and chest points.
- Return to the ear lobe and press along the entire spinal column, end on the sacral point as seen on the diagram above.
- Repeat the entire ear massage for one minute multiple times a day. This a simple way to be kind to yourself as you stimulate the feel good hormone, oxytocin with touch.

Individualized Therapy: Each person's ear acupressure treatment may vary based on specific health concerns and needs. Customize ear acupressure to target areas of imbalance and promote overall health and wellness.

Conclusion

In summary, ear acupressure leverages the microsystem of the ear to treat the entire body, offering a non-invasive and potentially effective approach to holistic health and wellbeing.

8

Nitric Oxide Dump

"Nitric Oxide Dump" refers to a specific exercise routine designed to naturally boost the production of nitric oxide in the body. Nitric oxide is a vital signaling molecule that plays numerous roles in cardiovascular health, immune function, nerve signaling, and other physiological processes.

What is Nitric Oxide?

Nitric Oxide is a gas that acts as a signaling molecule in the body. It is essential for various bodily functions, particularly in the cardiovascular, immune, and nervous systems. It helps regulate blood flow, blood pressure, and muscle contraction and is involved in nervous system communication and immune responses.

Benefits of Nitric Oxide for Endothelial Cells and Circulation

Vasodilation:

- Nitric oxide relaxes the smooth muscles in blood vessels, leading to vasodilation, which increases blood flow and reduces blood pressure.
- This effect helps maintain adequate oxygen and nutrient delivery to tissues and organs.

Endothelial Function:

- Nitric oxide plays a crucial role in maintaining the health of endothelial cells, which line the interior surface of blood vessels.
- It inhibits the adhesion of white blood cells and platelets to the endothelial cells, reducing inflammation and the risk of atherosclerosis (hardening of the arteries).

Anti-Thrombotic Effects:

- By preventing platelet aggregation (clumping), Nitric oxide reduces the risk of blood clots, which can lead to heart attacks and strokes.

Anti-Inflammatory Effects:

- Nitric oxide has anti-inflammatory properties that help protect blood vessels from damage and dysfunction.

Enhanced Exercise Performance:

- Improved blood flow and oxygen delivery to muscles can enhance exercise performance and reduce muscle fatigue.

The Nitric Oxide Dump by Dr. Zach Bush

See the 4 minute youtube workout in resources at the end of the book.

The "Nitric Oxide Dump" is a high-intensity exercise routine developed by Dr. Zach Bush. This exercise protocol is designed to stimulate the production and release of Nitric oxide in the large muscle groups, providing cardiovascular benefits and enhancing overall fitness. Here's a detailed look at the Nitric Oxide Dump exercise:

The Routine:

The routine consists of four simple exercises performed in quick succession:

- **Squats:** Stand with feet shoulder-width apart, squat down as if sitting in a chair, then return to the standing position. The arms come up as the weight goes back
- **Alternating Arm Raises:** Raise one arm straight up while lowering the other arm straight down, then switch arms in a controlled, alternating manner.
- **Arm Circles:** Extend arms straight out to the sides and make circles with the arms, first touching the sides of the hands in front of the body then swing arms over head touching the sides of the hands
- **Shoulder Presses:** Bend elbows and bring hands to shoulder height, then press arms upward until fully extended.

Repetitions and Sets:

- Perform each exercise for about 10-20 repetitions without rest between exercises.
- Complete three sets of the entire routine, with a brief rest period

between sets if needed.

Frequency:

- The Nitric Oxide Dump routine can be done two to three times a day, ideally spaced out to maximize Nitric oxide production throughout the day.

Benefits of the Nitric Oxide Dump Exercise

Increased Nitric Oxide Production:
The rapid activation of large muscle groups stimulates the endothelial cells in blood vessels to produce and release more Nitric oxide.

Improved Cardiovascular Health:
Regular practice can lead to improved blood flow, helps relax blood vessels, reduced blood pressure, and enhanced overall cardiovascular function.

Enhanced Exercise Efficiency:
The short duration and high intensity of the routine provide an efficient workout that can be easily incorporated into a busy schedule.

Increased Energy and Stamina:
The improved circulation and oxygen delivery to muscles can increase energy levels and stamina.

Improved Immune Function:
Nitric oxide plays a role in immune response by combating pathogens and supporting the body's defense mechanisms. Enhanced nitric oxide production may contribute to a stronger immune system.

Mood Enhancement:

Nitric oxide is involved in neurotransmission and mood regulation. Increased levels of nitric oxide may contribute to improved mood and mental wellbeing.

Increased Energy Levels:

The Nitric Oxide Dump exercises engage major muscle groups, promoting circulation and oxygenation. This can lead to increased energy levels and reduced feelings of fatigue and improved metabolic function.

Overall Wellbeing:

The routine promotes overall physical fitness and wellbeing, contributing to better health and quality of life.

Combining the Nitric Oxide Dump with a healthy diet, adequate hydration, and sufficient sleep can maximize its benefits for overall health and wellbeing.

Conclusion

If you struggle to find the time to work out, the Nitric Oxide Dump is a simple and effective exercise routine aimed at boosting Nitric oxide production in the body. By incorporating these exercises into your regular routine, you can potentially support cardiovascular health, enhance immune function, improve mood, and increase overall vitality. Always consult with a healthcare professional before starting any new exercise regimen, especially if you have pre-existing health conditions or concerns.

9

Gratitude

Gratitude is a powerful emotion and practice that has significant benefits for both physical and mental health. It also fosters a deep sense of connection with others and the universe. Let's delve into these aspects in detail:

Health Benefits of Gratitude

Mental Health Improvements:

- **Reduced Stress and Anxiety:** Practicing gratitude can lower levels of stress hormones and decrease anxiety.
- **Enhanced Mood**: Gratitude is linked to higher levels of positive emotions and overall happiness.
- **Depression Relief:** Regular gratitude practice can reduce symptoms of depression by shifting focus from negative to positive aspects of life.

Physical Health Benefits:

- **Improved Sleep:** People who practice gratitude tend to have better sleep quality and experience fewer sleep disturbances.
- **Boosted Immune System:** Grateful individuals often have a stronger immune response.
- **Reduced Pain:** Gratitude has been associated with lower levels of perceived pain and discomfort.

Social Benefits:

- **Stronger Relationships:** Expressing gratitude can strengthen bonds and improve relationships.
- **Increased Empathy:** Grateful individuals are more likely to exhibit prosocial behaviors and show empathy towards others.

Whole-Person Connection with Gratitude

Gratitude fosters a holistic sense of wellbeing by connecting different aspects of the self—mind, body, and spirit—with the world around us:

- **Connection with Others:** Gratitude enhances social connections and fosters a sense of belonging and community. By expressing gratitude, individuals build stronger, more supportive relationships.
- **Connection with the Self:** Gratitude encourages self-reflection and self-awareness, helping individuals recognize their own worth and appreciate their experiences.
- **Connection with the Universe:** Practicing gratitude can create a sense of spiritual connection and alignment with the larger universe, fostering a feeling of being part of something greater than oneself.

Two Branches of Gratefulness

Seeing everything as an opportunity:

- This branch of gratefulness involves viewing all experiences—positive and negative—as opportunities for growth and learning. It's about recognizing that every situation offers a chance to gain insight, develop resilience, and enhance personal development.
- Mindset Shift: By adopting this perspective, individuals shift their mindset from one of scarcity or negativity to one of abundance and possibility. This helps in maintaining a positive outlook even in challenging times.

Being thankful for that opportunity:

- This branch focuses on expressing thankfulness for the opportunities presented by various experiences. It's about actively acknowledging and appreciating the lessons, growth, and positive outcomes that arise from different situations.

Appreciation as the Easiest Emotion to Access

Active Appreciation: Practicing this form of gratitude involves consciously recognizing and expressing thanks for the opportunities that come your way, thus reinforcing a positive cycle of appreciation and acknowledgment.

Appreciation is considered one of the easiest emotions to access when shifting to a higher place on the emotional scale. Here's why:

- **Immediate and Tangible:** Appreciation can be easily felt by focusing on simple, immediate aspects of life, such as a beautiful sunset, a kind gesture, or a moment of peace.
- **Broad Applicability:** There is always something to appreciate, no matter how small. This makes it accessible in any situation.
- **Positive Feedback Loop:** Expressing appreciation often leads to more positive feelings and experiences, creating a reinforcing cycle of positive emotions.

Steps to Cultivate Appreciation

- **Mindful Observation:** Pay attention to the small, positive details in your daily life. Notice things that bring you joy or comfort, however minor they may seem.
- **Gratitude Journaling:** Write down things you appreciate each day. This practice helps to solidify the habit of noticing and valuing positive aspects of life. This is a great bedtime practice then start you day by reading your journal, setting an intention to find gratitude in this new day.
- **Expressing Thanks:** Verbally express appreciation to others. Whether it's a simple thank you or a heartfelt acknowledgment, expressing gratitude strengthens social bonds and reinforces positive feelings.

Whole-Person Connection through Gratitude and Appreciation

Practicing gratitude and appreciation can transform your overall well-being by:

- **Enhancing Emotional Resilience:** Helps you cope with stress and adversity by focusing on positive aspects and opportunities.
- **Fostering Spiritual Growth:** Deepens your connection to the universe and a higher power, promoting a sense of purpose and meaning.
- **Improving Physical Health:** Contributes to better sleep, a stronger immune system, and reduced pain and discomfort.
- **Strengthening Relationships:** Builds trust, empathy, and support in your relationships with others.

Conclusion

Consider starting your day with the "A Grateful Day Video" with David Steindl-Rast. This 5 minute video rewires appreciation in your being. See the URL in the resources at the end of the book.

Grounding in Gratitude is an combination of touch, breath, movement and focused attention on each chakra for mind-body-spirit (whole person) gratitude integration.

By incorporating gratitude and appreciation into your daily life, you can experience profound benefits across all aspects of your being, creating a more fulfilling, connected, and harmonious existence.

Grounding in Gratitude

- Sit or stand comfortably with feet grounded into the floor.
- Expand arms out to the sides with every inhale.
- With every exhale, place hands on a different region of the body and say the associated gratitude phrase:

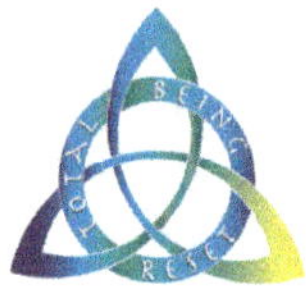

Inhale	Exhale	Say with exhale
Arms down by side	Hands on thighs	"I am rooted in gratitude"
Arms slightly higher than sides of chair	Hands below the navel	"I am balanced in gratitude"
Arms extended to just below a T	Hands to solar plexus	"I am empowered in gratitude"
Arms to a T	Hands to heart	"I feel gratitude"
Arms to just above a T	Hands to throat	"I speak gratitude"
Arms to a Y	Hands to eyebrows	"I see gratitude"
Arms above your head	Hands to top of head	"I am gratitude"

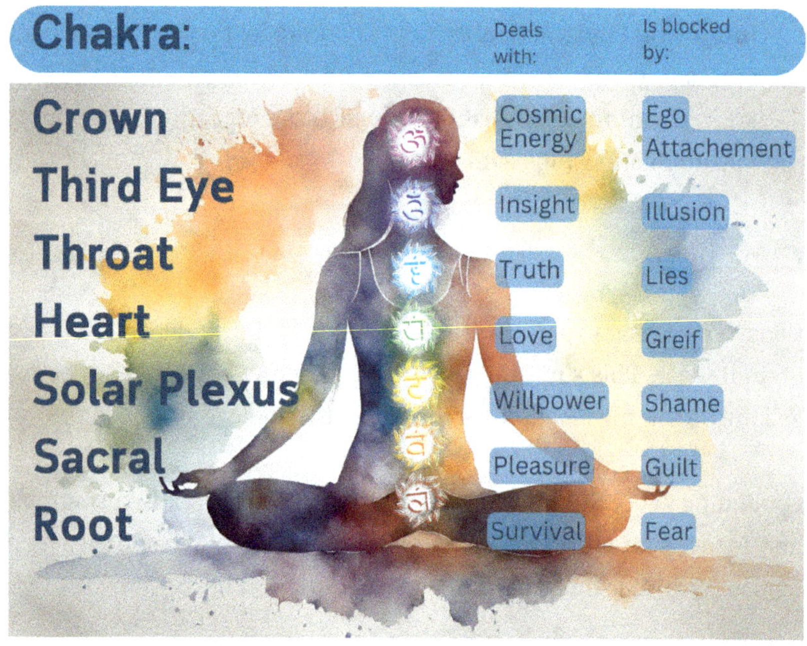

10

Loving Kindness Meditation

Loving Kindness Meditation, also known as Metta meditation, is a practice that involves cultivating an attitude of love and kindness towards oneself and others. The word "metta" is a Pali term that means benevolence, loving-kindness,and friendliness. This practice is rooted in Buddhist traditions but can be practiced by anyone regardless of religious affiliation.

The goal of loving kindness meditation is to develop compassion and unconditional positive regard for all beings, starting with oneself and gradually extending outward. This meditation practice typically involves repeating phrases that express good wishes towards oneself and others.

Benefits of Loving Kindness Meditation

The practice of metta meditation has numerous benefits, including:

Emotional Benefits:

- Increased Positive Emotions: Regular practice enhances feelings of joy, love, and gratitude.

- Reduced Negative Emotions: It helps diminish feelings of anger, resentment, and fear.
- Improved Self-Esteem: By cultivating self-love and compassion, individuals can improve their sense of self-worth. Kindness evolves from compassion into actively being kind to yourself.

Social Benefits:

- Enhanced Relationships: Practicing loving-kindness can improve relationships by fostering empathy and understanding.
- Greater Compassion: It encourages a compassionate outlook towards others, leading to more altruistic behaviors.

Health Benefits:

- Stress Reduction: It promotes relaxation and reduces stress.
- Improved Mental Health: It can help alleviate symptoms of depression and anxiety.
- Physical Health: Some studies suggest that it can have positive effects on physical health, such as reducing chronic pain and improving immune function.

Practicing Loving Kindness: Step-by-Step Guide

1. Start with Yourself:

Begin by finding a comfortable seated position. Close your eyes and take a few deep breaths to center yourself. Repeat the following phrases silently or aloud, directing the feelings of kindness and love towards yourself:

May I be safe and brave.
May I be happy.
May I be healthy.
May I live with ease.

2. Extend to Someone You Care About:

Next, think of someone you care about deeply. Visualize this person and repeat the phrases, sending them loving-kindness:
May you be safe and brave.
May you be happy.
May you be healthy.
May you live with ease.

3. Extend to a Stranger:

Now, bring to mind a neutral person, someone you don't have strong feelings about, such as a neighbor or someone you see regularly but don't know well. Send them the same wishes:
May you be safe and brave.
May you be happy.
May you be healthy.
May you live with ease.

4. Extend to a Someone who pushes your buttons:

Now, bring to mind a someone who triggers you, someone you have strong feelings about. In a non-judgmental way send them the same wishes:
May you be safe and brave.
May you be happy.

May you be healthy.

May you live with ease.

5. Extend to Your Community:

Broaden your focus to include your entire community or group of people you interact with regularly. This can be your workplace, social group, or local community:

May you be safe and brave.

May you be happy.

May you be healthy.

May you live with ease.

6. Extend to the World:

Finally, expand your focus to encompass all beings everywhere. Send loving-kindness to all life on the planet:

May you be safe and brave.

May you be happy.

May you be healthy.

May you live with ease.

Detailed Focus on Phrases

1. "May you be safe and brave":

- Safety: Wishing for protection from harm, both physical and emotional.
- Bravery: Encouraging courage to face challenges and adversities.

2. "May you be happy":

   - Focusing on the emotional wellbeing and joy of oneself and others.

3. "May you be healthy":

   - Encompassing physical, mental, and emotional health.

4. "May you live with ease":

   - Wishing for a life free from unnecessary stress and struggle, promoting peace and contentment.

Application of Phrases

For Self:

   - May I be safe and brave: Cultivate self-compassion, recognizing your own need for safety and courage.
   - May I be happy: Foster inner joy and contentment.
   - May I be healthy: Prioritize your own wellbeing.
   - May I live with ease: Strive for a balanced and peaceful life.

For Someone You Care About:

   - May you be safe and brave: Wish for their protection and courage.
   - May you be happy: Desire their joy and fulfillment.
   - May you be healthy: Hope for their overall wellbeing.

- May you live with ease: Wish for a smooth and stress-free life.

For a Stranger:

- May you be safe and brave: Extend kindness to those you don't know well.
- May you be happy: Foster a sense of connection and goodwill.
- May you be healthy: Wish for their health and wellness.
- May you live with ease: Desire ease and peace in their lives.

For Someone who Pushes Your Buttons:

- May you be safe and brave: Wish for their protection and courage
- May you be happy: Desire their joy and harmony
- May you be healthy: Hope for their overall physical, mental and emotional health
- May you live with ease: Wish for a smooth and stress-free life.

For Your Community:

- May you be safe and brave: Encourage a sense of safety and collective courage.
- May you be happy: Promote communal happiness and harmony.
- May you be healthy: Support the health of the community.
- May you live with ease: Strive for a peaceful and supportive environment.

For the World:

- May you be safe and brave: Send global wishes for safety and courage.
- May you be happy: Desire happiness for all beings.
- May you be healthy: Hope for the health and wellbeing of the planet.
- May you live with ease: Wish for a world free from suffering and filled with peace.

Conclusion

Loving Kindness meditation is a powerful practice for cultivating loving-kindness and compassion towards oneself and others. By systematically extending good wishes from oneself to others, it fosters a deep sense of interconnectedness and promotes emotional, social, and physical wellbeing.

11

Centering Prayer

Centering Prayer is a form of contemplative prayer or receptive meditation that focuses on deepening one's relationship with the Divine (or God, Source, etc.) through interior silence. It is rooted in the Christian mystical tradition but can be practiced by people of any or no specific faith background.

What is Centering Prayer?

Centering Prayer is a method of silent prayer that prepares us to receive the gift of contemplative prayer, in which we experience God's presence within us, closer than breathing, closer than thinking, closer than consciousness itself. This form of prayer is both a relationship with God and a discipline to foster that relationship.

How to Practice Centering Prayer

- **Choose a Sacred Word:** Select a word that symbolizes your intention to consent to God's presence and action within you. This word could be something like "peace," "love," "God," "amen," or any word that holds spiritual significance for you.
- **Find a Quiet Place:** Sit comfortably with your eyes closed, relax, and silently introduce the sacred word as the symbol of your consent to God's presence and action within.
- **Notice Thoughts, Feelings, and Sensations:** During the prayer, as you become aware of thoughts, feelings, emotions, or physical sensations, gently return to your sacred word. The goal is not to fight these thoughts or sensations but to acknowledge them and then let them go by returning to the sacred word.
- **Consistent Practice:** Centering Prayer is usually practiced for 20 minutes, twice a day. Consistency is key to deepening the practice and reaping its benefits.

Receptive Meditation

- **Noticing and Letting Go:** In Centering Prayer, you practice being receptive rather than directive. This means noticing thoughts, emotions, and physical sensations as they arise, but not engaging with them. Instead, you gently let them go by returning to your sacred word.
- **Deepening Presence:** The repeated act of returning to your sacred word cultivates a deepening presence and awareness of the divine within. This practice helps shift your focus from the incessant chatter of the mind to a deeper, more peaceful state of being.

Shifting Thoughts and Emotions

Centering Prayer teaches you to shift your focus from distractions to a place of inner stillness. This skill becomes invaluable in daily life as it helps you:

- **Manage Stress:** By practicing letting go of stressful thoughts and emotions during prayer, you can apply the same principle to stressful situations in daily life.
- **Enhance Emotional Regulation:** The practice of noticing and releasing thoughts and emotions fosters greater emotional regulation and resilience.
- **Cultivate Inner Peace:** Regular practice helps cultivate a sense of inner peace and groundedness that you can carry into your everyday interactions and decisions. The sacred word can act as a mantra through the day to reaffirm the connection with Source.

Emotional Evacuation and Release of the Ego Self

Emotional Evacuation: This term refers to the process of releasing pent-up emotions and psychological patterns that may be rooted in the unconscious mind. Through the practice of Centering Prayer, you create a space where these hidden emotions can surface and be gently released without attachment or judgment.

Release of the Ego Self: The ego self, or the false self, is the part of you that identifies with your thoughts, emotions, and sensory experiences. It is often driven by fear, desire, and a need for control. Centering Prayer facilitates the release of the ego self by:

- **Surrendering Control:** The practice teaches you to surrender control and let go of the need to manage or fix your thoughts and emotions, allowing a deeper, divine presence to emerge.

- **Embracing Humility:** It fosters humility by helping you recognize that you are not the center of your thoughts and emotions; instead, you become more attuned to a higher, more authentic self that is connected to the Divine.
- **Experiencing True Self:** As you release the ego self, you begin to experience your true self, which is grounded in love, peace, and unity with the divine source.

Benefits of Centering Prayer

- **Spiritual Growth:** Deepens your relationship with the Divine and fosters spiritual growth.
- **Emotional Healing:** Helps in emotional evacuation and healing by bringing unconscious emotions to the surface and releasing them.
- **Inner Peace:** Cultivates a sense of inner peace and wellbeing.
- **Improved Focus:** Enhances your ability to stay focused and present in the moment.

Conclusion

Being aware of the divine presence within you, the core of your being, or the universal light and connection inside you, gives you access to a deep source of wisdom and energy. This connection is lost when you see yourself as separate from the universe. By noticing your thoughts, emotions, and feelings, and then immediately shifting to a sacred word during meditation, you can strengthen your ability to make that shift in everyday life. My sacred word, "Awe," is used during my daily meditation, but it also serves as my moment-to-moment mantra to shift to gratitude, acceptance, and appreciation.

12

Ho'oponopono

Ho'oponopono is a Hawaiian practice of reconciliation and forgiveness. The word "ho'oponopono" translates to "to make right" or "to rectify an error." This practice is rooted in the belief that our external reality is a reflection of our internal state and that by healing ourselves, we can heal our relationships and experiences.

The Basic Principles of Ho'oponopono

Ho'oponopono operates on the principles of repentance, forgiveness, gratitude, and love. It involves a process of acknowledging and taking responsibility for the negative emotions or situations we encounter, seeking forgiveness, expressing gratitude, and reinforcing love.

The Traditional Phrases

The traditional Ho'oponopono prayer involves repeating the following four phrases:

- **I'm Sorry:** This phrase acknowledges that you recognize an issue or

problem exists and that you feel regret or sorrow for your part in it.
- **Please Forgive Me:** This phrase seeks forgiveness for any harm or negativity you have caused, whether consciously or unconsciously.
- **Thank You:** This phrase expresses gratitude for the opportunity to heal and for the forgiveness you are receiving.
- **I Love You:** This phrase reinforces the power of love and serves as a reminder of the interconnectedness of all things.

How to Practice Ho'oponopono

- **Identify the Issue:** Focus on a specific problem, emotion, or situation that you want to heal or address.
- **Repeat the Phrases:** Silently or aloud, repeat the traditional Ho'oponopono phrases: "I'm sorry. Please forgive me. Thank you. I love you."
- **Feel the Emotions:** As you repeat the phrases, allow yourself to truly feel the emotions associated with each one. This could mean feeling genuine regret, seeking forgiveness with an open heart, expressing sincere gratitude, and reinforcing the love you have.
- **Focus on the Healing:** Visualize the healing process taking place within you and extending outward to others involved in the situation.

Benefits of Ho'oponopono

- **Relief from Shame, Blame, and Guilt**: By practicing Ho'oponopono, individuals can release feelings of shame, blame, and guilt. The process of seeking and offering forgiveness helps to clear these depleting emotions and promote a sense of peace.
- **Improved Relationships:** The practice encourages taking responsibility for one's actions and emotions, which can lead to healthier, more harmonious relationships.

- **Emotional Healing:** Ho'oponopono facilitates emotional healing by addressing and releasing past traumas, regrets, and resentments.
- **Increased Self-Love and Acceptance:** Repeating the phrases "Thank you" and "I love you" can enhance feelings of self-love and acceptance, fostering a more positive self-image.
- **Enhanced Spiritual Connection:** The practice can deepen one's spiritual connection and sense of interconnectedness with others and the universe.
- **Stress Reduction:** By promoting forgiveness and letting go of negative emotions, Ho'oponopono can help reduce stress and promote a sense of inner calm.

Incorporating Ho'oponopono into Daily Life

Ho'oponopono can be practiced anytime, anywhere. It can be used in moments of distress, as part of a daily meditation or prayer routine, or whenever you feel the need to clear negative emotions and restore balance. By consistently practicing Ho'oponopono, individuals can cultivate a habit of forgiveness, gratitude, and love, leading to a more peaceful and fulfilling life.

Ho'oponopono is a powerful tool for personal transformation and healing. By embracing its principles and regularly practicing the prayer, individuals can experience profound emotional and spiritual benefits, creating a more harmonious and loving existence for themselves and those around them.

The adapted Ho'oponopono prayer provides a beautiful and expanded version of the traditional practice, incorporating elements of personal responsibility, ancestral healing, and gratitude. Here's a breakdown of each part of the adapted prayer and how it contributes to the overall practice:

Adapted Ho'oponopono Prayer Breakdown

"I am sorry, (name the emotion) for whatever in me creates this emotion."

- **Meaning:** This phrase acknowledges that you are taking responsibility for your emotions fueled by resistance and any internal factors that may be contributing to them. It recognizes that your thoughts, beliefs, and actions may play a role in the emotions you experience.
- **Purpose:** To cultivate self-awareness and accountability, and to express genuine remorse for any negativity within yourself.

"Forgive me, my family, my relatives, and my ancestors."

- **Meaning:** This phrase extends the request for forgiveness beyond yourself, including your family, relatives, and ancestors. It acknowledges that negative patterns and emotions can be passed down through generations.
- **Purpose:** To seek forgiveness not only for your own actions but also for any inherited or collective issues. This fosters a sense of collective healing and liberation from past burdens.

"Thank you for this opportunity to cleanse and let go."

- **Meaning:** This phrase expresses gratitude for the chance to heal and release negative emotions. It recognizes the importance of the healing process and appreciates the opportunity to grow and transform.
- **Purpose:** To foster an attitude of gratitude, which is essential for

emotional healing and wellbeing. Gratitude helps to shift the focus from the negative to the positive aspects of the healing journey.

"I love you for everything."

- **Meaning:** This phrase reinforces the power of love in the healing process. It expresses unconditional love for yourself, others, and the universe, acknowledging the interconnectedness of all beings.
- **Purpose:** To cultivate a deep sense of love and compassion, which are fundamental to personal and collective healing. Love helps to dissolve negative emotions and replace them with renewing, nurturing energy.

Practicing the Adapted Ho'oponopono Prayer

Breath deeply to center yourself. Consider using the relax, release, reset breathing practice

Identify the Emotion or Issue: Bring to mind the specific emotion, situation, or issue you want to address. Focus on it without judgment.

Repeat the Prayer: Silently or aloud, repeat the adapted Ho'oponopono prayer:
"I am sorry for whatever in me creates this emotion."
"Forgive me, my family, my relatives, and my ancestors."
"Thank you for this opportunity to cleanse and let go."
"I love you for everything."

Feel the Emotions: As you repeat the phrases, allow yourself to truly feel the associated emotions. Let the words resonate deeply within you. This is a necessary and powerful step in releasing stored emotions.

Visualize Healing: Visualize the negative emotions being released and replaced with healing light and love. Imagine this light spreading through you to every cell in your body and extending to your family, relatives, ancestors, and beyond.

Regular Practice: Incorporate this prayer into your daily routine or whenever you feel the need to address negative emotions. Consistent practice can deepen its impact and benefits.

Benefits of the Adapted Ho'oponopono Prayer

- **Emotional Release:** Helps to release feelings of shame, blame, and guilt by acknowledging and addressing their roots.
- **Ancestral Healing:** Recognizes and heals generational patterns and traumas, promoting collective wellbeing.
- **Self-Forgiveness and Compassion:** Fosters self-forgiveness and compassion, essential for personal growth and healing.
- **Gratitude and Love:** Cultivates gratitude and love, which are powerful emotions that enhance overall emotional and spiritual health.
- **Holistic Healing:** Addresses healing on multiple levels – personal, familial, and ancestral – leading to a more profound and holistic transformation.

The adapted Ho'oponopono prayer is a powerful tool for healing and transformation. It allows individuals to take responsibility for their emotions, seek forgiveness, express gratitude, and cultivate love. By incorporating this practice into your life, you can experience profound emotional and spiritual benefits, creating a more harmonious and fulfilling existence.

Conclusion

Ho'oponopono allows access to forgiveness in a unique way, without the need to retell the personal story, thus avoiding the triggering of past hurts. The practice leads to post traumatic growth and resilience by addressing the root cause of suffering, moral injury. Moral Injury is when someone feels they have violated their moral compass or conscience like participating in, witnessing, or failing to stop an act that goes against personal principal and moral values. Though we don't dive deeply into this topic in this book, it is an important part of healing. Since moral injury percolates in us a shame, blame, guilt, and resentment, rewiring of mind, body, and spirit is possible with Ho'oponopono.

13

Awe

Definition of Awe

Awe is a profound emotional experience characterized by a combination of wonder, reverence, and sometimes even fear or respect. It often arises when we encounter something vast, powerful, or beyond our ordinary understanding. Awe can inspire a sense of connectedness to something greater than ourselves, triggering feelings of humility and expanding our perspective.

Awe is a multifaceted emotion that can signal a complete immersion into the awe experiences with the sensation of goosebumps. Goosebump experiences relived the sights, sounds, taste, smell, tough and emotional tone of an experience that activates the ventral vagus nerve profoundly.

Resetting to an awe experience is an inner resource that creates renewing emotions to prevent the default mode network of the mind from replaying the energy depleting past or anticipated future experience. Just like Netflix streaming autoplay, you can get stuck continuing with the same thought patterns. Awe is like picking up the remote and stopping the show before the next episode starts; switching from a scary or emotionally draining show to a renewing, feel good flick. Awe can reset the mind, body and spirit simultaneously in a extraordinary way.

Awe arises from various sources, each offering a unique and profound experience. Whether it is through witnessing acts of moral beauty, participating in collective events, immersing in the wonders of nature, being moved by music, contemplating sacred geometry, experiencing the profound moments of birth and death, or having life-changing epiphanies, awe has the power to connect us to something greater than ourselves. This connection can inspire humility, gratitude, and a deeper appreciation for the world and our place within it.

Dacher Keltner's Research on Moral Beauty and Awe

Dacher Keltner, a prominent psychologist and professor at the University of California, Berkeley, has extensively studied emotions, including the experience of awe. His research highlights how moral beauty—acts of kindness, courage, and compassion—can be among the most profound and moving sources of awe.

Moral Beauty: A Profound Source of Awe

Definition: Moral beauty involves witnessing acts of great virtue, selflessness, and moral excellence. These acts can be characterized by exceptional kindness, bravery, compassion, and integrity.

Keltner's Findings:

- **Frequency and Intensity:** Keltner's research shows that experiences of awe frequently stem from observing moral beauty. These instances are often cited as some of the most intense and memorable experiences of awe.
- **Emotional Impact:** Witnessing moral beauty can deeply move individuals, evoking strong emotional responses such as tears, goosebumps, or an overwhelming sense of admiration and respect. These reactions highlight the profound impact that witnessing virtue can have on an observer.
- **Inspiration and Motivation:** Acts of moral beauty often inspire individuals to emulate these virtues in their own lives. Observing such acts can motivate people to engage in prosocial behaviors, increase their empathy, and foster a desire to contribute positively to their communities.
- **Connection and Unity:** Witnessing moral beauty can create a sense of connectedness and unity among individuals. It can break down barriers, fostering a sense of shared humanity and common values. This connection is a powerful antidote to feelings of isolation and division.

Examples of Moral Beauty

- **Altruism:** Acts of selfless giving, such as volunteering to help those in need or making significant personal sacrifices for the wellbeing of others.
- **Courage:** Witnessing individuals stand up against injustice, often at great personal risk, to protect others or to uphold ethical principles.
- **Compassion:** Observing acts of deep empathy and kindness, such as caring for the sick, comforting the grieving, or rescuing those in distress.

Implications of Keltner's Research

- **Mental and Emotional Health:** Experiences of awe, particularly from moral beauty, can have significant benefits for mental and emotional health. These experiences can reduce stress, increase feelings of wellbeing, and foster a more positive outlook on life.
- **Social Cohesion:** By highlighting the importance of moral beauty, Keltner's research suggests that encouraging and celebrating virtuous behavior can strengthen social bonds and promote a more compassionate and cohesive society.
- **Educational and Leadership Applications:** Understanding the impact of moral beauty can inform educational programs and leadership training. By teaching and modeling virtuous behavior, educators and leaders can inspire others and create environments that prioritize ethical conduct and compassion.

Moral Beauty Conclusion

Dacher Keltner's research underscores the profound nature of awe experiences derived from witnessing moral beauty. These moments not only deeply move individuals but also inspire positive change, foster social connection, and enhance overall wellbeing. By recognizing and celebrating acts of kindness, courage, and compassion, we can cultivate a more empathetic and unified society.

The Awe of Collective Effervescence

Definition: Collective effervescence is a concept introduced by the sociologist Émile Durkheim, referring to the energy, excitement, and sense of unity that people experience when they come together in a group, particularly during shared activities or rituals. This phenomenon can evoke a powerful sense of awe, as individuals feel like a part of something much larger than themselves.

Characteristics of Collective Effervescence

- **Sense of Unity:** When people participate in group activities such as religious ceremonies, concerts, sports events, or protests, they often feel a profound connection with others, transcending individual differences.
- **Heightened Emotions:** These gatherings can generate intense emotions, such as joy, excitement, and a sense of belonging, which are amplified by the shared experience.
- **Shared Purpose:** Engaging in a collective activity with a common goal or purpose can enhance the feeling of solidarity and collective identity, leading to a deeper emotional impact.
- **Transcendence:** Participants may feel they are part of a greater whole, experiencing a sense of transcendence that can be deeply moving and spiritually uplifting.

Examples of Collective Effervescence

- **Religious Gatherings:** Large-scale religious ceremonies or pilgrimages, where participants engage in rituals and shared worship, can create a powerful sense of communal spirituality and awe.
- **Music Festivals and Concerts:** The collective energy of a crowd enjoying live music can lead to an intense feeling of connection and exhilaration.
- **Sports Events:** Fans cheering for their team together can create a strong sense of unity and shared emotion, especially during moments of victory or defeat.

- **Social Movements and Protests:** Participating in demonstrations or movements for a common cause can evoke a profound sense of solidarity and purpose.

Benefits of Collective Effervescence

- **Emotional Wellbeing:** The shared positive emotions and sense of belonging can boost overall emotional wellbeing and reduce feelings of loneliness.
- **Strengthened Social Bonds:** These experiences can deepen social connections and foster a sense of community and mutual support.
- **Increased Cooperation and Altruism:** Feeling part of a larger group can encourage cooperative behavior and altruism, as individuals are more likely to prioritize collective wellbeing over individual interests.

Collective Effervescence Conclusion

Collective effervescence is a powerful source of awe that emerges from the shared experiences and emotions of being part of a group. It can foster a deep sense of connection, unity, and transcendence, enhancing emotional wellbeing and strengthening social bonds. By participating in group activities and rituals, individuals can experience the profound and uplifting impact of collective effervescence.

The Experience of Awe When Immersed in Nature

Definition: Awe in nature refers to the profound emotional experience people have when encountering the vastness, beauty, and complexity of the natural world. This type of awe often involves a mix of wonder, admiration, and a sense of connection to something greater than oneself.

Characteristics of Nature-Induced Awe

- **Vastness:** Encountering expansive landscapes, such as mountain ranges, oceans, or deserts, can evoke a sense of the immense scale and grandeur of nature.
- **Beauty:** The stunning visual appeal of natural elements, such as sunsets, forests, waterfalls, and wildlife, can inspire deep admiration and emotional uplift.
- **Complexity and Intricacy:** Observing the intricate details of natural phenomena, such as the delicate structure of a flower, the patterns in a spider's web, or the interconnectedness of an ecosystem, can lead to a sense of wonder and amazement.
- **Transcendence:** Being in nature often provides a feeling of being part of something larger and more timeless, fostering a sense of peace and spiritual connection.

Examples of Awe in Nature

- **Grand Landscapes:** Standing at the edge of the Grand Canyon, witnessing the vastness of the night sky in a dark-sky reserve, or viewing the Northern Lights can evoke awe.
- **Natural Events:** Experiencing a powerful thunderstorm, watching a solar eclipse, or observing a migration of animals can be deeply moving.

- **Everyday Natural Beauty:** Simple moments like watching the sunrise, hearing the sound of waves crashing on the shore, noticing a bee pollinating a flower or walking through a dense forest can also inspire awe.

Benefits of Nature-Induced Awe

- **Emotional Wellbeing:** Exposure to natural beauty can reduce stress, enhance mood, and promote feelings of happiness and tranquility.
- **Increased Connectedness:** Experiencing awe in nature can foster a greater sense of connection to the environment and encourage pro-environmental behavior.
- **Perspective Shifts:** Nature-induced awe can help put personal concerns into perspective, promoting a sense of humility and a broader understanding of one's place in the world.

Awe in Nature Conclusion

Experiencing awe in nature involves encountering the vastness, beauty, and complexity of the natural world. This type of awe can deeply move individuals, fostering emotional wellbeing, a sense of connectedness, and perspective shifts. By immersing ourselves in nature, people can access the profound and uplifting benefits of nature-induced awe.

The Experience of Musical Awe

Definition: Musical awe refers to the profound emotional reaction elicited by music, characterized by feelings of wonder, admiration, and deep emotional connection. This type of awe arises from the beauty, complexity, and emotional power of musical compositions and performances.

Characteristics of Musical Awe

- **Emotional Intensity:** Music has the power to evoke strong emotions, such as joy, sadness, exhilaration, or nostalgia. The depth of these emotional responses can lead to a sense of awe.
- **Complexity and Skill:** Witnessing the technical mastery and intricate composition of music can inspire awe. This includes the precision of musicians, the harmony of instruments, and the innovative use of musical elements.
- **Beauty:** The aesthetic appeal of music, including melody, harmony, rhythm, and dynamics, can captivate listeners and evoke a sense of wonder and admiration.
- **Transcendence:** Music can create moments of transcendence, where listeners feel transported beyond the ordinary, connecting deeply with the music and experiencing a sense of unity and timelessness.

Examples of Musical Awe

- **Live Performances:** Experiencing a powerful live performance by a skilled musician or orchestra can evoke awe, especially when the music creates a shared emotional experience among the audience.
- **Iconic Compositions:** Listening to masterpieces like Beethoven's Symphony No. 9, Mozart's Requiem, or contemporary works that push the boundaries of musical expression can inspire awe.
- **Innovative Music:** Encountering music that blends genres, uses innovative techniques, or features unique instrumentation can lead to a sense of wonder and admiration for the creativity and skill involved.
- **Personal Moments:** Hearing a song that resonates deeply with

personal experiences or emotions, or being moved by a piece of music in a significant moment, can evoke a powerful sense of awe.

Benefits of Musical Awe

- **Emotional Release and Connection:** Musical awe can facilitate emotional release, and helping listeners process and connect with their feelings. It can also create a sense of emotional connection with the performers and other listeners.
- **Enhanced Wellbeing:** The emotional uplift and transcendent experiences provided by music can improve overall wellbeing, reduce stress, and promote mental health.
- **Inspiration and Creativity:** Experiencing awe in music can inspire creativity and motivate individuals to engage with music more deeply, whether by creating their own music or exploring new genres.

Musical Awe Conclusion

Musical awe is a profound emotional experience characterized by deep admiration, emotional intensity, and a sense of transcendence. Whether through live performances, iconic compositions, innovative music, or personal moments, musical awe can evoke powerful emotions, enhance wellbeing, and inspire creativity. By engaging with music, individuals can access the transformative and uplifting power of musical awe.

Awe with Epiphany

Definition: An epiphany is a sudden, profound realization or insight that often comes unexpectedly and leads to a new understanding or perspective. Experiencing awe with an epiphany involves the sense of wonder and amazement that accompanies these moments of clarity and revelation.

Characteristics of Epiphany-Induced Awe

- **Sudden Insight:** Epiphanies occur abruptly, often when one is not actively seeking answers. This sudden clarity can be startling and deeply moving.
- **Transformative Understanding:** The insights gained during an epiphany can significantly change one's perspective, beliefs, or approach to life. This transformative quality adds to the sense of awe.
- **Emotional Impact:** The realization that comes with an epiphany often triggers strong emotional responses, such as joy, relief, or a sense of liberation, contributing to the feeling of awe.
- **Connection to Something Greater:** Epiphanies often provide a sense of connection to a larger truth or understanding, making individuals feel part of a greater whole and enhancing the feeling of awe.

Examples of Epiphany-Induced Awe

- **Personal Insights:** Realizing a profound truth about oneself, such as recognizing a long–held pattern of behavior or suddenly understanding one's purpose or passion.
- **Intellectual Breakthroughs:** Experiencing a moment of clarity that solves a complex problem or unifies previously disconnected pieces

of knowledge, often seen in scientific or creative fields.

- **Spiritual Revelations:** Having a deep spiritual or existential insight, such as a moment of enlightenment or a sudden understanding of a spiritual teaching.
- **Relational Epiphanies:** Gaining a new perspective on relationships, such as understanding the depth of someone's love or realizing the importance of forgiveness.

Benefits of Epiphany-Induced Awe

- **Personal Growth:** Epiphanies can lead to significant personal development and transformation, encouraging individuals to make positive changes in their lives.
- **Enhanced Wellbeing:** The emotional release and newfound understanding that come with an epiphany can improve mental and emotional wellbeing, providing a sense of peace and fulfillment.
- **Increased Creativity and Problem-Solving:** The insights gained during an epiphany can inspire new ideas and approaches, enhancing creativity and problem-solving abilities.
- **Strengthened Connection to Others and the Universe:** The sense of connection to larger truths or shared human experiences can foster empathy, compassion, and a deeper sense of unity with others and the world.

Epiphany-Induced Awe Conclusion

Awe with epiphany is a powerful experience characterized by sudden, transformative insights that evoke wonder, amazement, and deep emotional impact. These moments of clarity can lead to personal growth, enhanced wellbeing, increased creativity, and a stronger sense of connection to others and the universe. By remaining open to new experiences and perspectives, individuals can cultivate the potential for epiphany-induced awe and its profound benefits.

The Awe Experience Related to Birth

Definition: The awe experience related to birth encompasses the profound emotional and psychological reactions that arise during the process of childbirth and the emergence of new life. This type of awe is characterized by a mixture of wonder, reverence, and deep emotional connection.

Characteristics of Awe at Birth

- **Miracle of Life:** Witnessing the creation and arrival of a new life often evokes a sense of wonder and amazement at the complexity and beauty of the process of birth.
- **Emotional Intensity:** Birth is accompanied by powerful emotions such as joy, relief, love, and sometimes fear or anxiety. The intensity of these feelings contributes to the sense of awe.
- **Connection and Bonding:** The birth of a child fosters a profound sense of connection and bonding among parents, family members, and the newborn, enhancing the feeling of unity and love.
- **Transcendence:** The experience of birth often feels transcendent, as it touches on themes of creation, continuity of life, and the cycle of existence, making individuals feel part of something greater and timeless.

Examples of Awe at Birth

- **Childbirth:** Being present during the labor and delivery of a child, whether as a parent, family member, or medical professional, can evoke awe through the raw beauty and intensity of the experience. This goes beyond humans for those who have been there for any birth ranging from horses to sea turtle hatches.
- **First Moments:** Witnessing the first breaths, cries, and movements of a newborn, and the immediate bonding moments between the baby and parents, can be deeply moving and awe-inspiring.
- **Parental Experience:** For new parents, the realization of bringing a new life into the world, the sense of responsibility, and the overwhelming love for their child can be profound sources of awe.
- **Witnessing Growth:** Observing the rapid development and growth of a newborn over the initial days, weeks, and months, and marveling at the complex and miraculous process of life unfolding.

Benefits of Awe at Birth

- **Emotional Bonding:** The awe experienced during birth strengthens the emotional bonds between parents and their newborn, promoting attachment and fostering a loving family environment. Anyone witnessing a birth knows the heightened connection you feel with the newborn.
- **Enhanced Wellbeing:** The positive emotions and sense of wonder associated with birth can improve mental and emotional wellbeing, providing a deep sense of fulfillment and happiness.
- **Perspective Shift:** The experience of birth can lead to a broader perspective on life, emphasizing the importance of family, love, and the continuation of life, and often shifting priorities and values.
- **Increased Empathy and Compassion:** Witnessing or experiencing

the miracle of birth can enhance empathy and compassion towards others, recognizing the shared human experience and the preciousness of life.

Awe at Birth Conclusion

The awe experience related to birth is a profound and deeply emotional reaction to the miracle of new life. It encompasses intense emotions, a sense of connection and bonding, and a transcendent understanding of the cycle of life. The awe felt during birth can strengthen emotional bonds, enhance wellbeing, shift perspectives, and increase empathy and compassion, making it one of the most powerful and transformative experiences in human life.

The Experience of Awe as It Relates to Death

Definition: The experience of awe in relation to death involves profound emotional and existential reactions to the end of life. This type of awe is characterized by a mixture of reverence, mystery, and deep reflection on the nature of existence and mortality.

Characteristics of Awe at Death

- **Mystery and Transcendence:** Death often evokes a sense of mystery and the unknown, prompting deep contemplation about the nature of life, the afterlife, and the universe.
- **Emotional Intensity:** The emotions surrounding death are powerful and multifaceted, including grief, love, fear, and acceptance. The intensity of these feelings contributes to the awe experience.
- **Profound Reflection:** Encounters with death often lead to profound

reflections on one's own life, values, and priorities, fostering a greater appreciation for the present moment and the preciousness of life.

- **Connection and Continuity:** Death can evoke a sense of connection to something larger, whether through spiritual beliefs, the continuation of life through others, or the natural cycle of birth and death.

Examples of Awe at Death

- **Witnessing a Peaceful Passing:** Being present during the peaceful death of a loved one can evoke awe through the serenity and dignity of the process, and the deep emotional connections shared.
- **Cultural and Religious Rituals:** Participating in or observing death rituals and ceremonies, which often imbue the event with a sense of sacredness and communal reverence, can be awe-inspiring.
- **Natural Encounters with Death:** Observing the natural cycle of life and death in the environment, such as the changing seasons, the death of an old tree, or the end of an animal's life, can evoke a sense of awe at the continuity and balance of nature.
- **Personal Reflections on Mortality:** Moments of personal contemplation about one's own mortality, especially during significant life events or crises, can lead to an awe-inspiring realization of the fleeting nature of life and the importance of living meaningfully.

Benefits of Awe at Death

- **Perspective Shifts:** Contemplating death can lead to significant shifts in perspective, encouraging individuals to live more authentically, prioritize what truly matters, and cherish their relationships and experiences.
- **Increased Empathy and Compassion:** Encounters with death can

deepen empathy and compassion for others, recognizing the shared human experience of loss and the need for support and understanding.

- **Emotional Healing and Acceptance:** Experiencing awe in the context of death can facilitate emotional healing and acceptance, helping individuals to process grief and find peace with the natural cycle of life.
- **Spiritual Growth:** For many, encounters with death inspire spiritual growth and a deeper connection to their beliefs, fostering a sense of comfort and continuity beyond physical existence.

Awe at Death Conclusion

The experience of awe as it relates to death is a profound emotional and existential reaction to the end of life. It encompasses deep emotions, reflections on mortality, and a sense of connection and transcendence. This type of awe can lead to perspective shifts, increased empathy, emotional healing, and spiritual growth, making it a deeply transformative and meaningful aspect of the human experience.

The Experience of Awe as It Relates to Sacred Geometry

Experiencing awe at seeing sacred geometry in the physical world around us can be a deeply profound and transformative experience. Sacred geometry refers to geometric patterns and shapes that hold symbolic and spiritual significance across various cultures and traditions. These patterns are often found in nature, architecture, art, and even within the human body, reflecting a universal harmony and order.

Examples of Sacred Geometry in the Physical World

Natural Patterns:

- **Fibonacci Sequence:** Found in sunflowers, pinecones, and nautilus shells, the Fibonacci sequence is a mathematical pattern where each number is the sum of the two preceding ones (0, 1, 1, 2, 3, 5, 8, 13, …).
- **Golden Ratio:** Also known as Phi (φ), the Golden Ratio is approximately 1.618 and is observed in the proportions of the human body, seashells, and the architecture of ancient civilizations.

Geometric Shapes:

- **Mandala:** A spiritual and ritual symbol in Hinduism and Buddhism, mandalas are intricate geometric designs representing the cosmos. They are used for meditation and as a tool for focusing attention inward.
- **Platonic Solids:** These five geometric shapes (tetrahedron, cube, octahedron, dodecahedron, icosahedron) are named after the ancient Greek philosopher Plato and are believed to correspond to the elements of nature.

Experiencing Awe in Sacred Geometry

When encountering sacred geometry in the physical world, people often report feelings of awe, wonder, and reverence. Here's how this experience unfolds:

- **Perception of Order and Harmony:** Sacred geometry reflects a deep sense of order and harmony in the universe. Witnessing these patterns can evoke a profound sense of connection to something greater than oneself.

- **Spiritual and Symbolic Meaning:** Many cultures attribute spiritual and symbolic meanings to sacred geometry. For example, the Flower of Life symbolizes creation and the interconnectedness of all life.
- **Emotional Impact:** Awe at seeing sacred geometry can elicit emotional responses such as joy, peace, and a deep appreciation for the beauty and complexity of existence.

Integration into Daily Life

- **Mindfulness Practice:** Incorporate mindfulness techniques to notice and appreciate sacred geometry in your surroundings. Take moments to observe patterns in nature, architecture, or artwork.
- **Creative Expression:** Engage in creative activities such as drawing, painting, or crafting geometric designs. This process can deepen your understanding and connection to sacred geometry.
- **Contemplation and Meditation:** Use sacred geometry as a focal point for contemplation or meditation. Reflect on its meaning and how it resonates with your spiritual or philosophical beliefs.

Sacred Geometry Conclusion

Experiencing awe at seeing sacred geometry in the physical world offers an opportunity for spiritual growth, creativity, and a deeper understanding of universal principles. Whether in natural formations, architectural wonders, or artistic expressions, these geometric patterns invite us to contemplate the mysteries of existence and our place within it. Embrace these moments of awe with openness and reverence, allowing them to inspire and uplift your daily life.

Review of Awe

Awe is a profound emotional experience characterized by a combination of wonder, reverence, and sometimes even fear or respect. It often arises when we encounter something vast, powerful, or beyond our ordinary understanding. Awe can inspire a sense of connectedness to something greater than ourselves, triggering feelings of humility and expanding our perspective.

Conclusion

Awe is a multifaceted emotion that can arise from various sources, each offering a unique and profound experience. Whether it is through witnessing acts of moral beauty, participating in collective events, immersing in the wonders of nature, being moved by music, contemplating sacred geometry, experiencing the profound moments of birth and death, or having life-changing epiphanies, awe has the power to connect us to something greater than ourselves. This connection can inspire humility, gratitude, and a deeper appreciation for the world and our place within it.

14

Total Being Reset Conclusion

Creating a daily routine that incorporates various practices intermittently can be highly beneficial for enhancing overall wellbeing, emotional balance, and spiritual growth.

Here's how you can structure such a routine:

Daily Routine Incorporating Various Practices

Morning Routine:

- Breathwork (5-10 minutes):

- Start with a simple deep breathing exercise such as relax, release, rest breathing or alternate nostril breathing to oxygenate the body, calm the mind, and prepare for the day.

- HeartMath Biofeedback (5-10 minutes):

- Use a HeartMath device or app to practice coherence breathing. Focus on heart-centered breathing while visualizing positive emotions like gratitude or love. This helps to synchronize heart rate variability and promote emotional balance.

- Loving-Kindness Meditation (10-15 minutes):

- Cultivate compassion and loving-kindness towards yourself and others. Repeat phrases such as "May I be safe and brave. May I be happy. May I be healthy. May I live with ease." while visualizing sending love and kindness to yourself and others.

- Nitric oxide dump

- End your shower with 1-2 minutes of cold water

- Watch A Grateful Day Video (see resources for link)

Midday Routine:
  - Giggle, laugh, hum, dance, sing and hug frequently

- Awe Experience (Awe Walk) (15-30 minutes):

- Take a walk outdoors in nature or a serene environment. Engage your senses fully and notice the beauty and wonder around you. Allow yourself to feel awe and gratitude for the natural world.

- Gratitude Practice (5-10 minutes):

- Keep a gratitude journal or simply reflect on three things you're grateful for today. Do the Grounding in Gratitude practice. This practice helps shift focus towards positive aspects of life and fosters a sense of contentment and appreciation.

Evening Routine:
  - **Centering Prayer (10-20 minutes):**

  · Engage in silent prayer or meditation focused on contemplative silence and connection with the divine. Use a sacred word or phrase to gently bring your mind back to center when distractions arise.

- **Yoga Nitric Oxide Dump (10-15 minutes):**

  · Practice a short sequence of yoga asanas or the Nitric Oxide Dump exercises to release tension, improve flexibility, and promote circulation. These movements also stimulate the release of nitric oxide, benefiting overall cardiovascular health.

- **Sound Healing or Ear Acupressure (10-15 minutes):**

  · End your day with a session of sound healing using crystal bowls or Tibetan singing bowls. Alternatively, perform ear acupressure by gently massaging or pressing specific points on the outer ear to promote relaxation and balance energy flow.

Additional Practices Throughout the Day:
  - **Emotional Freedom Technique (EFT):**

  · Use EFT tapping as needed throughout the day to address stress, anxiety, or emotional triggers. Focus on specific issues or emotions and tap on the meridian points while repeating affirmations.

- **Ho'oponopono:**

  · Practice the Ho'oponopono prayer whenever you encounter challenging emotions or conflicts. Repeat the phrases "I'm sorry, please forgive me, thank you, I love you" or the adapted phrases to release negative feelings and restore inner peace.

Tips for Success:

- **Consistency:** Aim to practice these techniques consistently each day to maximize their benefits. Start with a manageable duration and gradually increase as you become more comfortable.
- **Integration:** Integrate these practices into your existing daily routines. For example, incorporate breathwork and gratitude practice into your morning routine, and centering prayer and yoga into your evening routine. Most of the short strategies take only a minute to insert before or after meeting or sending emails.
- **Adaptation:** Modify the routine based on your personal preferences, schedule, and specific needs. Experiment with different techniques and adjust as necessary to find what works best for you.

By incorporating these various practices into your daily routine, you can cultivate a holistic approach to health and wellbeing, promoting emotional resilience, spiritual connection, and overall vitality.

Embracing these practices with dedication and consistency, you can develop resilience within yourself and also within your community and the broader universe. The overlapping benefits of attunement, appreciation, awe, abundance, acceptance, and allowing—all cultivated through daily practice—contribute to a thriving individual who resets to be a light of joy and bliss. This journey of self-discovery and healing nurtures our heart-mind-body connection with kindness and compassion. Somatic practices as well as Ho'oponopono release the body's stored blame shame and guilt making it easier to avoid behaviors and habits like addiction and self abuse.

The integration and layering of the multiple practices listed allow for integration of the entire human system as a whole. Yoga, movement and vagus nerve activation are truly antidotes to the chronic stress states that evolve into chronic inflammation, decreased immune function and lifestyle diseases.

Research across cultures regarding ancient practices validates the integration of these practices for maximum benefit. Cortisol, our stress hormone, stays in our system for 12 hours and keeps pumping when we are in a chronic perceived stress state and dosing with oxytocin, DHEA, gaba and Nitric oxide through these practices is the antidote. These thrive neurochemicals are short lived, lasting 1-2 hours. Setting up a daily calendar of self kindness practice is a simple and effective way to counter perceived threat and flourish in an internal space of attunement (heart coherence), appreciation, awe, abundance, acceptance. These A's overlap and grow together with daily practice to develop a resilient person in a resilient community and a resilient universe.

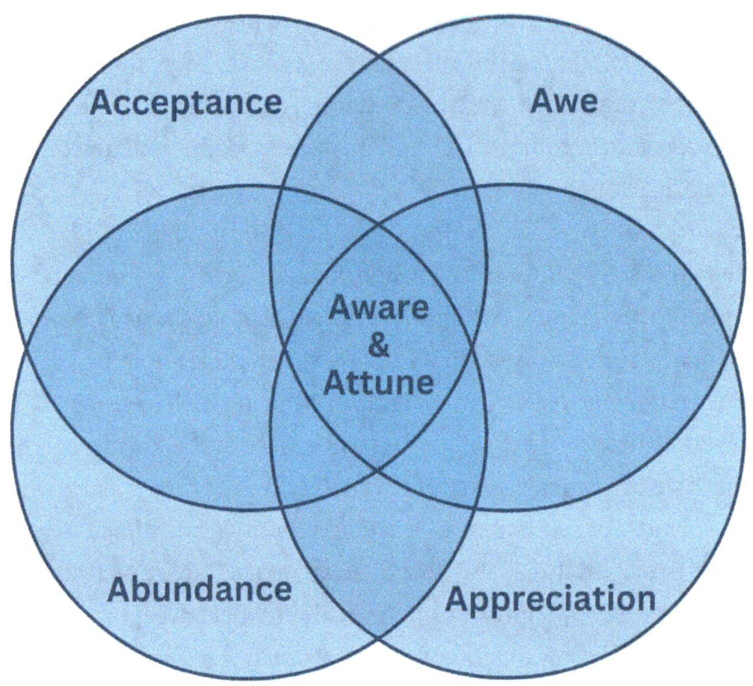

Acceptance
Awe
Aware
&
Attune
Abundance
Appreciation

15

Resources

Emerson, D., & Hopper, E., PhD. (2012). *Overcoming Trauma through Yoga: Reclaiming Your Body.* North Atlantic Books.

Grateful Living. (2017, August 22). *A Grateful Day with Brother David Steindl-Rast - Gratefulness.org* [Video]. YouTube. https://www.youtube.com/watch?v=zSt7k_q_qRU

Grateful Living. (2024, June 13). *Welcome to grateful living.* Grateful.org. https://grateful.org/

HeartMath. (2024, June 27). HeartMath. https://www.heartmath.com/

HeartMath Institute. (n.d.). *HeartMath Institute.* https://www.heartmath.org/

HELPTALKS. (2019, September 16). *HELP TALK: Ho'oponopono Healing by Dr. Karishma Ahuja* [Video]. YouTube. https://www.youtube.com/watch?v=al-ardSUZns

Karam, A., Van Der Braak, A., Aluli, M., & Mai, M. M. K. K. P. (2022). *Transformative spiritualities: for the pilgrimage of justice and peace.* https://doi.org/10.58863/20.500.12424/4171024

Keating, T. (2023). *Open Mind, Open Heart 20th Anniversary Edition.* Bloomsbury Publishing.

Keltner, D. (2009). *Born to be Good: The Science of a Meaningful Life.* W. W. Norton & Company.

Keltner, D. (2024). *Awe: The New Science of Everyday Wonder and How It Can Transform Your Life.* Penguin.

Louv, R. (2013). *Last Child in the Woods: Saving our Children from Nature-Deficit Disorder.* Atlantic Books Ltd.

Newman, L., PhD. (2024, June 17). *Accredited EFT Tapping Training with EFT International.* EFT International. https://eftinternational.org/

Oleson, T. (2013). *Auriculotherapy manual: Chinese and Western Systems of Ear Acupuncture.* Elsevier Health Sciences.

Salzberg, S. (2019). *Real Happiness, 10th Anniversary Edition: A 28-Day Program to Realize the Power of Meditation, Enhanced Version.* Workman Publishing Company.

Salzberg, S. (2020). *Real change: Mindfulness to Heal Ourselves and the World.* Flatiron Books.

Steindl-Rast, D., Schwartzberg, L., & Carlson, P. (2013). *A good day: A Gift of Gratitude.* Union Square & Co.

Sutton, J., PhD. (2024, May 23). *Polyvagal theory explained (& 18 exercises & resources)*. PositivePsychology.com. https://positivepsychology.com/polyvagal-theory/

Tgpnq. (2020, September 14). *Myofacial release - Innate Vitality.* Innate Vitality. https://innatevitality.net.au/myofacial-release/

What is Sound Healing - the Sound Healing Academy. (n.d.). https://www.academyofsoundhealing.com/what-is-sound-healing

ZachBushMD. (2017, September 5). *ZACH BUSH MD | 4 minute workout* [Video]. YouTube. https://www.youtube.com/watch?v=PwJCJToQmps

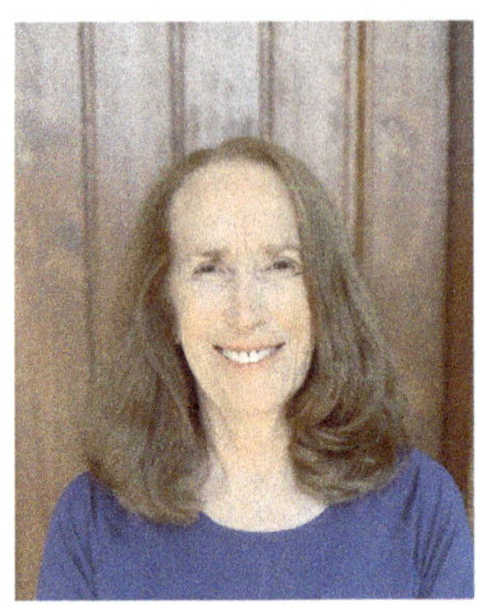

About the Author

Dr Christine OBrien DO is an Osteopathic Primary Care Physician who has vast experience in the integration of mind, body, and spirit as a yoga instructor, acupuncturist, centering prayer, and mindfulness-based stress reduction meditation teacher, sound healer, and Heartmath trainer. Her passion is to facilitate finding the reset practices that integrate into daily life with ease and purpose for each individual. She spent the past 15 years honing these skills while working with veterans, as the director of Whole Health at the Cheyenne VA. As the mother of seven children, she approaches Total Being Resets with utmost kindness for yourself and others. She is dedicated to the healing power of nature to cultivate awareness of Wonder and Awe to shift into resilience and connection. Christine's unique style of integrating body-based practices for vagus nerve activation is profound yet simple.

You can connect with me on:

🌐 https://www.totalbeingreset.com